SpringerBriefs in Well-Being and Quality of Life Research

For further volumes:
http://www.springer.com/series/10150

Thomas E. Jordan

Quality of Life and Mortality Among Children

Historical Perspectives

Springer

Thomas E. Jordan
University of Missouri
University Blvd. 1
St. Louis, MO 63121
USA

ISSN 2211-7644 ISSN 2211-7652 (electronic)
ISBN 978-94-007-4389-2 ISBN 978-94-007-4390-8 (eBook)
DOI 10.1007/978-94-007-4390-8
Springer Dordrecht Heidelberg New York London

Library of Congress Control Number: 2012938005

Printed on acid-free paper

Springer is part of Springer Science+Business Media (www.springer.com)

Preface

The purpose of this study is to investigate the personal and numerical aspects of death among children across three centuries. *Quality of Life* is the construct used to explore the complex. For nineteenth century England and Wales, and Ireland, it is formulated as two national measures, the VICQUAL and QUALEIRE indexes. Each index consists of several domains containing relevant numerical data. For the seventeenth and eighteenth centuries written sources—diaries, essays, inscriptions, poems, and church records, for example, are employed. In addition to limited numerical materials from that era, attention is drawn to the reaction of parents to the death of a child, and to the variety of ways in which the loss was reacted to, and memorialized.

Contents

Introduction

Among people engaged in the pursuit of children's welfare emphasis is placed on the opportunities childhood presents through its plasticity for character formation and acquisition of skills. To be sure, infancy is seen as a delicate transition from the security of the uterus to the independence with vulnerability of the early stages; but for those weeks there is recourse to modern medicine in most cases, and optimism is the value which prevails. The early years are construed as an opportunity to counter the effects of unhealthy environments in a community or family. Such benign outcomes are endorsed by religious and secular people around the world. Within this consensus there is room for local and sectarian values as people transmit selected elements of the local culture.

Largely absent from this scenario in the modern world is the death of children; medicine, science, and philanthropy, plus governments and public policy, address opportunities for bettering the lives of children, especially the youngest. In recent decades poliomyelitis was banished from the Western scene and, worldwide, smallpox is no longer the rite of childhood whose survivors bore the marks of its violence. The death of many children tends to be an event reported from places around the world which are far away, although tragedies can appear closer to home from time to time.

Nineteenth century data from England and Ireland demonstrate that the concept, quality of life, provides a useful approach for understanding mortality among children in the Victorian era. England and Wales had centers of industrialization with a sorry list of disamenities (Williamson 1982). Ireland was still largely agricultural, although Belfast and the Lagan valley increasingly resembled towns across the Irish Sea, in England and Scotland.

A substantial difference was the earlier aggregation of social data in England and Wales, while Ireland did not begin to gather vital statistics until 1863–1864. The censuses of Ireland conformed to the pattern in England and Wales, a step which facilitates comparisons in some areas. However, mortality data from Victorian Ireland did not meet the quality level attained on the larger island, so that explorations and comparisons in child mortality are less satisfactory. When children die families mourn their loss privately, and public discourse does not address the singularity of the family's trauma. However, the Sudden Death syndrome (SIDS) is now recognized in public discourse, and sends ripples beyond parents and siblings which touch relatives, friends, and the general public. In that sense, the death of a child through SIDS becomes a public event.

Mourning the deaths of children evokes awareness of their futures eclipsed by an unknowable agenda. Recently, a newspaper gave an account of a woman whose son was stillborn 20 years before. She had named the child, and periodically she initiates a make-believe conversation with him. At age twenty or so she imagines what his life might have been up to that point. A Victorian lady wrote that memory of a stillbirth had not left her long after the event, and she memorialized the child in a poem many years later.

In still earlier days, when the death of children was even more frequent, loss of one child after another led to extended periods of mourning. This may account in part for the impression of the early modern period as one of persisting depression. In eras burdened by economic and political problems stress was compounded by the experience of personal tragedy. There is the anecdote of the man who observed with bravado that he still had a Baker's dozen of surviving children, his need to compensate is evident, and suggests that grief takes many forms, at times posing the stark choice of whether to laugh or to cry—or to do both.

Modes of inquiry. The sources for consideration of mortality among children are diverse, and require a range of approaches. For today's information, and for archives as far back as the early nineteenth century, censuses at intervals of a decade are informative. For such sources research uses number as the data language or idiom of inquiry. Statistical procedures applied to numbers can identify effects and associations in data sets. Typical variables of interest whose influence is the question at hand are gender, age, and elements of peoples' social background. In this work census data also provide numerically based indexes of quality of life to explore data on mortality among children in the nineteenth century.

One measure of quality of life, is the VICQUAL index; it comprises fourteen factors in four domains. The second is the QUALEIRE index of quality of life in Ireland composed of fourteen elements in three domains. Connecting the two censuses is their similarity of format and procedure, although the two indexes are drawn from separate societies.

When research into children's mortality goes to a still earlier era the mode of inquiry becomes less number-centered. Sources are less likely to be numeric, and inquiry is more speculative. The investigator brings values to the procedures and sifts materials for relevance. Source materials include diaries, memoirs, and contemporary accounts—all of which provide content filtered through the outlook of two people, the investigator and the authors of documents.

The sources of that kind employed here include seventeenth century parish registers. They recorded christenings, marriages, and burials, and also the daily matters of paying bills to repair the church roof and to pay for candles. Occasionally we encounter a waspish note which might, on further consideration, have seemed un-charitable to the clerk who made the entry. For quality of life in the seventeenth century we make gross discriminations about peoples' way of life and its quality, and infer that they were rich or poor. An indicant of urban social quality of life is the number of hearths or windows counted in a dwelling, and on which taxation was based. The premise is that those with considerable amenities enjoyed a superior quality of life.

Insightful in a different way are the diaries and memoirs left to us by people who usually did not intend their jottings for public display. In this category is the diary of Samuel Pepys whose daily experiences in seventeenth century London, including his moral lapses, were set down in code. Pepys's account of the Great Fire of London in 1666, has validity derived from his personal role at the time. An empirical frame of mind was evident in the seventeenth century physician who sought to study the progress of influenza and related symptoms; he made the rounds of city churches and counted the number of coughs and sneezes.

Subjectivity inherent in scrutiny of personal documents is an example of a mode of inquiry which is complementary to seemingly objective and scientific methods. Both methods are employed when sources are varied and return us to a world long vanished. Against the claim of objectivity we evaluate statistical results as estimates within a degree of error. To admittedly subjective evaluations of documentary evidence we ascribe honesty of intent modulated by the values which the diarist brought to the task. In the case of John Aubrey's *Brief Lives*, set down in the seventeenth century, the validity of his little sketches is strengthened by his personal ties and leavened by his taste for gossip.

In this study of mortality among children from the seventeenth to the nineteenth century materials are subjective and objective opening up harsh realities as we seek to understand the life cycle and its entrances and exits.

My thanks to Ms. Helen E. Thorington who typed the manuscript; also my boundless thanks to Mr. Brad. Bomanz.

Thomas E. Jordan

Chapter 1
Mortality

The discipline of human development—known to some as *Auxology*—tends to be a dynamic enterprise; that is, it deals with the course of growth in living persons after conception, and the stages of that process are approached as temporary and evolving. The temporal aspect is extended when data sets are assembled from an earlier era in order to examine the interaction of social and natural forces on various aspects of development. For example, economic historians have found it useful to employ height and body mass as outcome variables when examining economic change. The heights of males during the Civil War in the United States, and British males and females during the Industrial Revolution are examples (Jordan 1993a, b).

The life cycle has a beginning and an end; whether in a former age or our own the process eventually reaches asymptote. Such an ending is generally associated with the later decades of life, and archives of vital statistics record the final event. Quite different, however, is the impact of death long before actuaries' projected end. In the young we see an interrupted course and unfulfilled promise. The premature end of life in the young was much more common in eras before our own; until the twentieth century, survival rather than death was the exception.

The reality of death among the young is improbable among our generation, and it receives scant attention among students of human development. The topic is more likely to arouse demographers. And yet in the human cycle the death of children constitutes a developmental measure. It becomes a criterion in the life cycle, but one with, as it were, a negative valence. Mortality as a criterion can structure inquiry as readily as height, weight, or cognitive attainment. It can, for example, serve as a dichotomous criterion in a multivariate design.

In this work the anti-criterion of death among children is used in two ways. The first is in the subjective idiom of anecdotes and documentary accounts of the deaths of children in eras well before our own. The second way uses number as the data language to explore the connection between deaths and the prevailing quality of life in the nineteenth century. This idiom can be traced to research on London's

T. E. Jordan, *Quality of Life and Mortality Among Children*,
SpringerBriefs in Well-Being and Quality of Life Research,
DOI: 10.1007/978-94-007-4390-8_1,

Bills of Mortality published in 1662 by John Graunt (assisted to a degree by Sir William Petty). The careful gathering, recording, and aggregation of data in civil archives of births and deaths and in decadal censuses express themes urged in the nineteenth century by the little known but influential Jeremy Bentham, and pursued by the physicians John Simon and William Farr.

The first locus in the numerical studies is England and Wales, and the second is Ireland. The two sites provide differing contexts. England and Wales, a statutary combination, was a place enduring the social strains and heavy price of industrialization. Ireland, in contrast, was a largely rural society with several modest urban centers. Ireland at mid-century endured the loss of the potato crop on a massive scale, an event which led to a loss of population by death and emigration, and to fundamental changes as a nation.

In consideration of children's deaths in an idiom beyond individual instances data sets are available as far back as the nineteenth century. In that era civil registration of births and deaths became systematic, although causes of deaths and age at the time of death and other useful pieces of information were initially lacking. When natural disaster struck, than as now, specific items of information tended to be slighted when matters more urgent than record-keeping concerns prevailed.

Sources for group data exist in censuses and public records. However, survival of such information has not been universal, and fire and war have destroyed valuable records. Dublin is an example of a city where records have been lost and found; Ireland's civil war led to loss of public archives in 1922. However, the Parish Records Society of Dublin, two decades earlier, had begun transcription of parish registers in a process still active today. In England, Ireland, and Sweden, for example, church and civil records have allowed reconstitution of family data on births and deaths.

Understanding death among children requires an estimate of the quality of life in the society into which they were born. In this study data are retrieved from census and similar sources, and they form quantitative estimates within which mortality records are considered. The overall hypothesis of this essay is that children's mortality can be understood within a framework of information which estimates the quality of life concurrent with the annualized death rates for the two sites, England and Wales and Ireland.

1.1 Death

To assess the scope of death young children it is helpful to examine early twenty-first century data. When examining mortality data from centuries before our own, a sense of the modern situation provides perspective.

In 2007 mortality for all boys and girls under one year of age (0–364 days) was 684.50 per 100,000 infants. This frequency dropped sharply in older age groups; in the 1–4-year group the rate was 28.60, followed by rates in the next older age segment of 13.70 deaths per 100,000 among 5–9-year olds. At these ages death was more likely among boys than girls. In 2007, the causes of death were, in order, "prematurity and low birth weight—a condition markedly higher among "non-Hispanic Black" infants. The second most frequent cause of death was "Maternal complications of pregnancy," followed by "complications of placenta, cord and membrane." The fourth and fifth causes of death were "respiratory distress" and "bacterial sepsis" (Xu et al. 2010).

In understanding the end of life, a corollary or reciprocal is the amount of life foregone by death in the earliest period of life. Death at one year, according to official statistics in 2007, ended a life expectancy of 77.50 years; within this generalization boys at 74.90 years of anticipated life fall below girls whose life expectancy is 79.90 years. For children born in 2010, the projected life span is 78.30 years; boys' life expectancy is 75.70 years, and for girls it is 80.80 years (Deaths … 2010). Around the world, according to the Organization for Economic Cooperation and Development (OECD 2011), three countries have the highest life expectancy; they are Japan and Switzerland at 82 years, followed by Italy where life expectancy is slightly lower. The bottom three countries are South Africa, India, and the Russian Federation. In contrast to these OECD findings, in mid-nineteenth century Dublin a child fortunate enough to reach the first birthday enjoyed the prospect of living until the early twenties. Today, United States' census data project the probability of living for a further 58.80 years.

It is apparent that today's children in the modernized world enjoy a far greater prospect of surviving infancy. Beyond that stage of development they have a long life expectancy—excepting comparatively infrequent hazards beyond the powers of pediatric medicine. With a grasp of our comparatively benign climate for child development, the scope of conditions in earlier times can be appreciated. To that end, an empirical formulation of quality of life can put into perspective the high mortality rates in the nineteenth century. Consideration of child mortality in England and Wales examines the facts in a social context of industrialization and political ferment. In the case of Ireland, child mortality among the very young is examined in a largely rural society with several urban centers all of which had just undergone the trauma of the Famine.

In the case of mortality data from England and Wales, after 1838, data are fairly plentiful. Incidence figures for children in the first year of life, in the age segment 0–4, and 5–9 years will be examined. In the case of Ireland, civil registration did not begin until 1864; from that era data on mortality under one year of age is extant.

However, the death of children amounts to more than comparative statistics. Death was an all too familiar event long before numbers became the data language of record. Families endured their losses and occasionally put words on paper to record their personal tragedy. Such accounts exist in memoirs, diaries, poetry, and other media. Anne Bradstreet mourned the death of a grandchild by invoking a theme of the era; namely, that infants and small children were God's provenance and were with their families on a temporary basis. She wrote,

> Farewell fair flower that for a space was lent,
> Then t'aen away unto Eternity (Illick 1975).

John Milton wrote that, "Young Lycidas is dead, ere his prime … who would not sing for Lycidas?" We now move to accounts of the death of children encountered in a range of sources, places, and times. The consideration begins a generation or so before Milton commemorated the loss of Edward King in the Irish Sea.

References

Jordan, T. E. (1993a). "L'Homme Moyen": Estimating the quality of life for British adults 1815–1914, an index. *Social Indicators Research, 29*, 183–203.

Jordan, T. E. (1993b). *The degeneracy crisis and victorian youth*. Albany: State University of New York Press.

Xu, J. et al. (2010). Deaths: Final data for 2007. National Vital Statistics Reports, 58. No. 19.

OECD. (2011). *Compendium of OECD well-being indicators*. Paris.

Illick, J. (1975). Child-rearing in seventeenth century England and America. In L. deMause (Ed.), *The history of childhood*. New York: Harper.

Chapter 2
Quality of Life

2.1 Introduction

The concept, *quality of life*, has several formulations. There is the personal, ever-changing perception one's life and its rewards and vicissitudes. Structured by emotions from pleasure to pain, and extending into past and future, the subjective version is dynamic and changeable. This perceived state is a sense of one's personal world which includes people, events, and the unpredictable. Despite its apparent solipsism personal quality of life is assessable through psychometric questionnaires.

The alternative formulation addresses society as a whole through lists of factors external to the individual, but impinging on the person directly or indirectly. A degree of detachment from the individual and an empirical flavor permit an objective estimate of quality of life in a particular place, and for a particular aggregate of people; the locus of inquiry may be a household, a neighborhood, a country, or a region, and the people will be a group of interest. These observations are summarized in the "… generic definitions of Quality of Life …" set forth by the Australian Center on Quality of Life in 2010:

> Quality of life is both objective and subjective. Each of these two axes comprises several domains which, together, define the total construct. Objective domains are measures through culturally relevant indices of objective well-being. Subjective domains are measured through questions of satisfaction.

Objective formulations of quality of life begin with the subjectivity inherent in the act choosing what to study by empirical means. The horizon is wide and includes choices about which people, places, occasions, and institutions to consider. Natural forces also enter, and can range from the amount of rain a place receives to the impact of earthquakes, tsunamis, hurricanes, and droughts. The subjective and objective can be combined; in the research of Pine et al. (1997),

T. E. Jordan, *Quality of Life and Mortality Among Children*,
SpringerBriefs in Well-Being and Quality of Life Research,
DOI: 10.1007/978-94-007-4390-8_2, © The Author(s) 2012

psychiatric states and obesity in the young were combined; this study also includes points in time.

The scope of quality of life has several aspects conveying a person's degree of internal to external focus. At one extreme is the examination of satisfaction with life (Diener et al. 1985); at the other is the use of quality of life as a concept to guide development of a nation; an example is Latvia (Karnitis 2006). Such aspirations call for well-honed specifics. For people dwelling in cities Wills-Herrera, Islam, and Hamilton (2009) formulated a thirteen-item schema for appraising subjective quality of life; the elements are:

Standard of living	Health	Future security	Health
Economic situation	Safety	Social conditions	Government
Local security	Business	Environment	Achievements
Sense of community	Relationships		

It is unlikely that respondents would rate all aspects of their lives as equally satisfactory. Such a predictable imbalance led Lyubomirsky et al. (2005) to ask, "Does happiness lead to success?" The question might be expanded to ask, "and for how many?" Related is the question of whether a high quality of life is attainable for an entire country. The Good Society Framework (ISQOLS 2010) set forth nine domains as a "comprehensive model of wellbeing."

Relationships	Peace and security	Environment and infrastructure
Economy	Culture and leisure	Spirituality and philosophy
Governance	Education	Health

Similarly, Cummins et al. (2005) reported a list of criteria for evaluating "The World's Best Country," drawn up by Lazakekic:

Income	Health	Freedom	Unemployment
Family life	Climate	Security	Gender equality
Political stability	Family and community		

There are commonalities in the three lists just presented, and there are unique items; also, there are elements which rise and fall in salience; political stability and security, for example, may not be reconcilable in some contexts.

The formulation of quality of life used by the Organization for Economic and Social Development (OECD 2011) in its survey of thirty-four countries explained how the concept influences lives:

> Quality of life defined as the set of non-monetary attributes of individuals, shapes their opportunities and life chances, and has intrinsic value under different cultures and contexts.

The concept is framed empirically through eight domains; they are:

> Quality status, work and life balance, education and skills, social connections, civic engagement and governance, environmental quality, personal security, subjective well-being.

OECD added four sustaining elements designated as *natural capital, economic capital, human capital, and social capital.*

It does not follow that what distinguishes quality of life for people as a whole automatically applies to individuals. Working within the framework of the British Household Panel Survey Plagnol and Scott (2011) asked individuals to tell them,

> … what things you consider are important for your own quality of life?

Respondents gave items within the following categories:

Health	Family	Finance	Happiness
Friends	Leisure	Home comforts	Employment
Misc. other	Freedom	Time self	Other material
Education	Other personal	Spiritual	Environment
Negatives (i.e., need more/better)			

The author concluded that perceptions of quality of life were likely to change when people experienced events such as marriage or the birth of a child. The life course rather than belonging to an age cohort explained changes associated with age.

The formulations of quality of life, so far, apply to the present day. There arises the search or quality of life in former times. In the case of the former Soviet Union, Brainerd (2010) sought answers in six cities from St. Petersburg in the north to Kharkov in what is now Ukraine. Of critical significance were periods in the new Economic Policy 1921–1928, and the era of rapid industrialization in 1929–1940. On a smaller scale, and in an earlier era, Lindberg (2009) examined the social and economic factors which led to the decline of two ports of the Hanseatic League, Danzig, and Lubeck.

Keeping records was well established in the German city, Breslau, in the seventeenth century allowing Edmund Halley (1693) to publish his "… Estimate of the Degrees of Mortality …" London's Bills of Mortality were the source of John Graunt's (1662) monograph on patterns of death by age and place. Interesting physical accounts from south county Dublin were transcribed by Flatman (1989). In this essay, two estimates of quality of life in the nineteenth century are employed. The VICQUAL index (Jordan 1993a, b) is applied to study children's mortality in Victorian England and Wales, and the QUALEIRE index (Jordan 2000) is applied to Ireland in the same century.

There arises the matter of what quality of life for children entails. In the seventeenth century, a colleague of Halley and Graunt, Sir William Petty, faced the challenge to arrange a superior quality of life for his young brother. After much of what he termed ratiocination (i.e., an interior dialog), Petty concluded that the best thing to do was to, "Let Nature work, and let him follow his own inclination (and) provide him a course of life whereby he may make the best use of his natural wares." For his two sons Petty provided a list of books to prepare them for their futures. In this work, quality of life for children is formulated as,

> The extent to which children can fulfill their potentials for self-realization and happiness in surroundings conducive to health and harmony.

This formulation reflects, of course, present-day perspectives. Applied literally to earlier times it seems quite inappropriate because children's role tended to be prescribed narrowly. Childhood itself was brief, and adolescence was not a clearly marked phase. By the teens young people were expected to function as adults, in some respects. For example, marriage viewed as a mechanism for the expeditious transfer of property and wealth. Family life was rough and tumble, and abuse of alcohol by parents placed children at risk for survival. For children without parents the future was bleak, at best. In the earliest days they lived or died on the streets. Depending on the ideology of the parish Vestry children might be put out to board; one Irish parish required that a boarded-out infant be presented alive every three months in order to continue welfare payments. Charles Dickens gave us Pip, and Dickens recalled the harsh terms of his early experience in a small factory. In the face of abuse of children which could be seen every day, the Victorians summoned the initiatives of Mary Carpenter and the oratory of Lord Shaftesbury, "The Children's Friend." In Ireland Edmund Rice and Richard Whately, for example, worked to improve the quality of life for children.

We view childhood and mortality from our own century and a perspective is necessary. Death itself was a denial of the elements proposed in the formulation of quality of life presented here; and it suggests the scope of mortality's impact among the young of earlier generations eliminating their *self-realization … happiness … health … harmony.*

References

Brainerd, E. (2010). Reassessing the standard of living in the Soviet Union: An analysis using archival and anthropometric data. *Journal of Economic History*, *70*, 83–117.

Cummins, R. A., Stokes, M., Michalos, A., Vitterso, J., Steel, P., Oberstrom, E., & Clay, N. (2005). The world's best country by Laza Kekic: A critique. *SINET*, *81*(1–4), 11.

Diener, E., Emmons, R. A., Larsen, R. J., & Griffin, S. (1985). The satisfaction with life scale. *Journal of Personality Assessment, 49*, 71–75.

Graunt, J. (1662). *Natural and Political Observations Mentioned in a Following Index, and Made Upon the Bills of Mortality*. London. Martin, Allestry, and Dicas.

ISQOLS, (2010). *The Good Society Framework*. Berlin.

Jordan, T. E. (1993a). "L'Homme Moyen": Estimating the quality of life for British adults, 1815–1914, an index. *Social Indicators Research, 29*, 183–203.

Jordan, T. E. (1993b). *The Degeneracy Crisis and Victorian Youth*. Albany, NY: State University of New York Press.

Jordan, T. E. (2000). The quality of life in Victorian Ireland, 1831–1901. *New Hibernia Review, 4*, 103–121.

Karnitis, E. (2006). Increasing quality of life as a goal for development of Latvia. *Applied Research in Quality of Life, 1*, 125–138.

Lindberg, E. (2009). Club goods and inefficient institutions; why Danzig and Lubeck failed in the early modern period. *Economic History Review, 62*, 604–628.

Lyubomirsky, S., King, L., & Diener, E. (2005). The benefits of frequent positive affect: Does happiness lead to success? *Psychological Bulletin, 131*, 803–855.

OECD. (2011). *Compendium of OECD Well-Being Indicators*. Paris.

Pine, D. S., Cohen, P., & Brook, J. (1997). Psychiatric symptoms in adolescence as predictors of obesity in early adulthood: A longitudinal study. *American Journal of Public Health, 87*, 1303–1310.

Plagnol, A. C., & Scott, J. (2011). What matters for wellbeing: Individual perceptions of quality of life before and after important life events. *Applied Research in Quality of Life, 6*, 115–138.

Wills-Herrera, E., Islam, G., & Hamilton, M. (2009). Subjective well-being in cities: A multidimensional concept of individual, social, and cultural variables. *Applied Research in Quality of Life, 4*, 201–221.

Chapter 3
Death of Children in the Sixteenth to Nineteenth Centuries

3.1 Introduction

From then to now: a sense of the present has assets and liabilities. The present is a world of the familiar in which the customs of the day are fairly well understood, and the actions and attitudes of people can be deciphered, although with exceptions. We interact with people and find in the flow of their lives echoes of our own experience. Our shared course through life is not without hazards or limits although the cycle can be extended by the technology of today's medicine. Today people tend to live on the premise that their sense of today will prevail and that living will extend without bounds.

In this chapter my hope is to construct an impression of an earlier world outlook, or sensibility, in which the course of life was interrupted frequently. It was experienced in the immediacy of new life, that of children, whose untimely deaths denied expression of their unique qualities and potentials.

There has been a tendency to project an indifference to the death of children onto parents in eras before our own. The mind-set of parents recorded in various writings does not support that canard for, despite their familiarity with death within the family circle, parents mourned each lost child. A less secular view of reality allowed bereaved parents a leavening measure of consolation. Of course, within that generalization are individual differences and cultural practices. They extend from the religious in which a child entered a spiritual world down to a pragmatic sense; in that valuation, a newborn might be enrolled in several insurance clubs so that a predictable hazard might be put to good use by hedging one's bet, as it were. The quality of life for infants was mediated in a calculus of risks and possibilities unique to each time and place. In this chapter some of these elements are elucidated from centuries past.

T. E. Jordan, *Quality of Life and Mortality Among Children*,
SpringerBriefs in Well-Being and Quality of Life Research,
DOI: 10.1007/978-94-007-4390-8_3, © The Author(s) 2012

3.2 Sources

Current approaches to quality of life postulate that the concept in its many formulations (e.g., Jordan 2010a–c) applies to the world of the living. Empiricism leads demographers to the edge of the grave and there they consider rates of mortality, etiology, and location. Such numbers appraise quality of life by, for example, evaluating comparative rates of death within a particular population.

When we attempt to recreate quality of life in former times the challenge is to access appropriate data; unlike searches in the twenty-first century, inquiry before the nineteenth century cannot draw on established databases such as the nineteenth century censuses of England and Wales, and of Ireland's thirty-two counties. There are caches of information from the seventeenth century in the form of numerical estimates of population but, for example, some are derived from calculating ratios of hearths per family, and estimates of persons per family. Occasionally, country churches yield information as at Colyton, Devon, (Sharpe 2002; Wrigley 1968), and Magherafelt, County Derry; from the latter, Morgan (1974) identified an increase of children dying before their third birthday, every 3–4 years.

There is material of unquestionable validity in the diaries and journals kept by figures such as Samuel Pepys (1633–1703) and John Evelyn (1620–1706), and the *Brief Lives* compiled by John Aubrey (1626–1697) are informative. Colonial England—e.g., Virginia—provided data on child deaths in the form of inscriptions in churchyards (Coffman 2009). With other Middle Atlantic colonies the region lost close to one-third by age 20 years. Eastern Maryland experienced a smallpox panic in 1737 (Smith 1980). The life expectancy of those born in Maryland was 20.80 years, and for immigrants to Maryland it was only 17.40 years (Kunitz 1984). Of course, for those who survived the early perilous years of life often extended into the late forties.

3.3 Death

In the earliest years addressed here thoughtful people reflected on the transience of life, and the cesura which surrounded them. Ordinary people experienced death frequently burying children, wives and husbands, and parents, and undertaking the rites of interment at frequent intervals. During times of plague such experiences were magnified, and entire families were wiped out. Plague struck London in 1603, 1625, 1636, and 1665 (Mullett 1938).

In this atmosphere of familiarity with death reflective people sometimes set down their thoughts in an epistolary form. In the county of Suffolk, c.1658, a number of burial urns containing Roman remains were unearthed. Reflecting on, "What time the persons of these ossuaries entered the famous Nations of the dead, and slept with Princes and Counsellors …" Sir Thomas Browne (1605–1682) concluded that death is, "the heaviest stone that melancholy can throw at a man … we live by an invisible sun within us … there is no opium against time … concluding,' tis all one to lie in St. Innocent's church-yard as in the sands of Egypt."

Browne presented his essay in a time and place when religion was all-present and secularism was unknown. There was a thin stream of intellectual thought arising from the writings of Sir Francis Bacon, Lord Verulam (1561–1626), which would in time subvert the universality of religious thought (Jardine and Silverthorne 2000). In the seventeenth century a few men in several countries contributed to the works of "natural philosophy," the field of endeavor we know as science. However, at the time the enterprise consisted merely of the works of a few brilliant men working in comparative isolation, but often in parallel. In optics, for example, there were Christopher Huygens and Anton van Leeuwenhoek in Holland, while Robert Hooke invented his tiny microscope in England. The Royal Society established by Charles II in 1662 became a medium for their correspondence.

Natural philosophers worked within a culture in which religious beliefs were active. For all but a few skeptics, the death of children and adults was a moment of transition into another life. Sir William Petty (Jordan 2007, 2010a–c), empiricist, statistician, and entrepreneur, included an avowal of the Anglican church in his many writings on population and other subjects. In his will, written a few years before his death in 1687, Petty declared, "I dye in the profession of that faith, and in the practice of such worship, as I find establht (sic) by the Law of my country … I willingly resigne my soul into His hands …" Such was the religious ferment in England that the era is marked by the profusion of Protestant sects. The 1640s and 1650s were replete with Anabaptists, Quakers, Ranters, Levellers, and Muggletonians—groups labeled as Independents (Hill 1975). The last Muggletonian appears to have died in the 1990s.

Yet Petty was an empirical investigator who played a role in the eventual differentiation of religion and science; the larger cultural complex included fairies, witchcraft, magic, and alchemy, so that the emerging science struggled to throw off a burden of muddled thinking and entrenched beliefs. Respect for authority which equated inquiry with impudence was a continuous hindrance to a slowly developing empiricism among the small band of natural philosophers.

Death was recorded in the seventeenth century in relatively informal ways. Law required that deaths be recorded and published in the Bills of Mortality; but the data entered there were gathered, in London and Dublin, by the searchers. They were to be, according to the precepts issued in London, "two sober Ancient Woemen, honest and discrete, within everye pish (sic) … which shalbe (sic) sworne trulye to search and make viewe of the bodye of anye … that they maye make true reporte to the Clarke of the parish …" (Forbes 1974). Illustrations of the era show them wearing tall pointed hats and carrying a long pole. Such elderly women rarely encountered a physician who could offer an explanation of the death, and they relied on the opinion of whoever was at hand. Given the state of medicine at the time, whose diagnoses included "planet-struck" and "the rising of

Table 3.1 Yearly bills of mortality

London			Dublin	
Anno	Burials	Births	Burials	Births
1680	21053	12747	1826	1096
1679	21730	12288	1397	1061
1678	20678	12601	1401	1045
1674	21201	11851	2106	942
1672	18230	12563	1436	987
1668	17278	11633	1699	1026
(Total)	120170	73683	9865	6157

the lights," the possibilities for error were great when recording deaths. However, it is clear that for a long time recorded deaths exceeded recorded births—a fact compromised by the presumption that births recorded equaled children born. "Observator"—Petty—summarized deaths and births in London and Dublin are shown in Table 3.1.

Hidden within the statistics of death was a problem which persists into the twenty-first century; it is violence toward children. There is a long tradition which has said "spare the rod and spoil the child". The adage invokes Scripture, and led to attempts to build character, but it also masks direct abuse leading to the death of children in all centuries.

At first glance the number of deaths at all ages in both Dublin and London should have left those centers of population quite empty; the explanation is that immigration from the provinces and hinterlands remedied the deficit. Within the numbers given for deaths we can be sure that they included children. Petty calculated the number of survivors by age in his 1672 book, *The Political Anatomy of Ireland* (Petty 1691). From birth to age six a cohort of 991 newborns declined to 704 survivors—a loss of 287 children. To age sixteen a further 242 children died, for a total of 529 out of the original 991 births. Absent from such calculations is the number of deaths in utero. The proportion of lost conceptions is hard to examine even today.

However, the 1700s provide information on children's deaths in the form of entries in diaries and anecdotes. In January 1658, the diarist, and future Fellow of the Royal Society, John Evelyn, recorded the death of his gifted son Dick who had reached age 5 years a mere 3 days before. "At 2 yeare and a halfe old he could perfectly reade any of the English, Latine, French (sic) or Gottic letters; pronouncing the three first languages exactly… and had a strange passion for Greeke … and had a wonderfull disposition to Mathematics …"

Death was not done with Mr. and Mrs. Evelyn; one month later, the diarist recorded, "The afflicting hand of God being still upon us, it pleased him also to take away from us this morning my other youngest sonn George now 7 weekes languishing at Nurse, breeding Teeth, and ending in a Dropsie: Gods holy will be don: he was buried in Deptford Church the 17th following …"

In 1670, Evelyn's friend, Sir William Petty (Jordan 2007), and his wife, Lady Elizabeth Waller Fenton Petty, lost two children to smallpox. The boy was named John, and the girl appears to have been an infant; possibly this last child was a chrysom—an unbaptized and so unnamed child. The Petty's suffered a third loss in the death of Lady Petty's son William, whose father was Elizabeth Waller's first husband, Sir Maurice Fenton. Petty's friend in his later years was Dr. William Molyneux; he and his wife lost three children. The diarist Samuel Pepys (1602–1603) was the fifth child and the first to survive in a group of seven offspring (Thrower 2003). Pepys and his wife Elizabeth de St. Michel were childless. Six of eight children of James II's first wife, Anne Hyde, died; the survivors were Mary and Anne. Later, none of the ten children of James 11s second wife, Maria D'Este, survived. The essayist Michel de Montaigne recorded, "I have lost two or three children in their infancy, not without regret, but without great sorrow" (Aries 1962).

A source of information about the death of children in the seventeenth century is the set of archives of Dublin parish churches reconstructed in the twentieth century. In the Victorian era, an interment in 1669 was opened at the north Dublin church of St. Michan and revealed, "… a pathetic baby corpse, from whose plump wrists still hand the faded white ribbons of its funeral … the very finger and toe nails of the child are still distinct." (Berry 1907). At the time, civic governance was managed by a Council and Mayor, and by the respective parishes which carried out a number of social functions. In 1624 St. John the Evangelist parish "paid for the burial of Besswoods daughters childe…. Besswoods sonne" (Mills 1906). In 1651 St. John's parish buried "Captain Mitchell & 4 children," victims, perhaps of the 1650 plague. In 1659 the vestry of the parish of St. Catherine and St. James paid for the funeral of the "orfant" daughter of John Yeates who was being raised by Luke Lowther. Sometimes a foster child had to be presented alive to a skeptical vestry for funding to continue. In the parish of St. Michan, on the north side of the river Liffey, in April 1698, the vestry interred, "a poor woman (sic) and a poor child, left in the church yard, whose names are not known." A month later, the parish buried "a child called Mary Sherin, the mother went away and left her" (Berry 1909). Six days later, the parish orphan, Mary Smithfield, nursed by Ann Hutton, was interred. A curiosity is that about this time, parish records began to note exactly where a corpse was interred—"in the third vault on the left hand, in the chancel, of this church of St. Michans" (Gillespie 2004).

In the child deaths considered so far the range of social classes has been broad, and death came to children of all classes whatever their quality of life, although social conditions increased the risk for the poor. From Sharpe's (2002) information from Colyton, Devon, by my count amounting to 8,277 live births, I have calculated the incidence of deaths for children by social level. The premise is that the social level of occupations connotes the material quality of life. The Colyton children were born across two centuries, 1600–1799. For the entire group the incidence of deaths in the under 5 years group is 20.33%. There is an inverse relationship between social level—fathers' occupational group—and child mortality. The series is as follows:

Group	Size	Deaths (%)
Gentry	1,204	16.60
Crafts	1,051	19.40
Laborers	653	22.40
Poor	1,491	27.57

The incidence of child mortality among the poor is one-half more than the incidence among the gentry over the two centuries. That discrepancy still persists today where public policy and practice are negligent.

Common to all classes was the risk posed to mothers by childbirth although, as Lewis (1998) pointed out, tuberculosis was probably a more certain risk. Being a "Great Ladie" conferred no immunity to women in labor; being one of that privileged class did not reduce their risk of mortality. From Lewis's data from 334 Great Ladies I calculate the mean death rate for the years 1600–1699 at 5.39%. Presumably it was at least as high, and probably higher, for their less favored sisters. Death associated with childbirth was always threatening to mothers. Approaching her next delivery Anne Dudley Bradstreet, who left Northampton for Salem, Massachusetts in 1630, composed a poem to her husband; she noted,

How soon, my dear, death may my steps attend,
How soon't may be they lot to lose thy Friend ...

Apart from its intrinsic merit the survival of women in labor protected children through the transmission of maternal antibodies to certain potentially fatal diseases (Landers 1987). Pervasive was the problem of hygiene, both personal and public. Great wealth was no protection from filth and vectors of disease. In his diary for 4 January 1665, Samuel Pepys (hardly a model of cleanliness) recorded that he, "... to My Lord of Oxford's ... and Lord help us ! so rude a dirty family I never saw in my life" (Le Gallienne 2003).

Around 1670, John Aubrey gave an account of how children were raised, "from the time of Erasmus till about 20 years past. The Gentry and the Citizens had little learning of any kind, and their way of breeding up their children was suitable to the rest: for whereas ones child should be ones nearest Friend, and the time of growing-up should be most indulged, they were as severe with their children as their schoolmaster.... The child perfectly loathed the sight of his parents as the slave his Torturor" (Dick 1949).

Giving birth was ill-understood; in his *Brief Lives*, John Aubrey traced the delivery of the political philosopher Thomas Hobbes on April 5, 1588 recording that, "His mother fell in labour with him upon the fright of the Invasion of the Spaniards" (Dick 1949). Such a view was reasonable at the time; the world outlook of ordinary people saw implications for uterine development, including death, in shock, and bad news. They were credulous and had no alternate to correct views held since time immemorial about life and death. The death of children was an event which while distressing was not unanticipated.

3.4 Health and Development

Understanding the death of children in eras long before our own begins with an appreciation of the state of society. Health of a population reflects the circumstance of life and its quality at the time. In the case of seventeenth century in Ireland and England the climate was cold—an era now referred to as the Little Ice Age; in January 1684 John Evelyn recorded that the Thames froze, and commerce flourished on the ice for several weeks. The corollary was that the poor suffered and common winter diseases flourished. Ireland also felt the cold, and both countries endured social chills which were near-fatal. In the case of England and Ireland political convulsions and war approached at the end of the 1630s. In England, the devious Charles the First began the 1640s increasing tension with Parliament; in time this degenerated into the two phases of the Civil War, and the eventual execution of the King. In Ireland, an uprising began in Ulster in 1641 beginning a decade of violence which ended with Oliver Cromwell's invasion in 1649. The social consequences for human development and welfare were serious. To use a phrase of the era—the world was turned upside down.

Not the least consequence was the impact on health for children and adults. At the best of times maintaining good health was a challenge among ordinary people. Personal hygiene was abysmal; the gorgeously dressed gentlemen at court used corners and closets as toilets. In his diary for 23 January 1669, Samuel Pepys recorded, "So to my wife's chamber … she finds out that I am lousy, having found in my head and body about twenty lice, little and great …" (Le Gallienne 2003).

Not surprisingly people in Ireland suffered from "the Irish ague," which we know as typhus. Smallpox was a hazard that children had to experience in the seventeenth century. John Evelyn, no stranger to worry about the health of his children, recorded in January 1684 that his daughter Susan "had some few small pox come forth on her … the small pox being very fatal;" fortunately, Susan Evelyn survived, as the astronomer Johannes Kepler had done before her; in his case the sequelae included myopia and double-vision (Hawking 2002). It may be noted in passing that in his autobiography Benjamin Franklin recorded the death from smallpox of his son at about age 4 years. Landers (1987) estimated smallpox deaths as 6.53% of all deaths in the later decades of the seventeenth century.

For all ages tuberculosis in two forms, glandular and pulmonary, was a threat to life; and scarlet fever was a virulent, often fatal disease—unlike the milder form into which it mutated in the nineteenth century. Malaria was endemic and killed several great men; an example is Henry Ireton, Cromwell's proconsul in Ireland, and Cromwell himself probably died of the disease. In England, in the counties of Essex and Kent near the Thames estuary, children were reported by visitors as of sallow complexion, with swollen bellies, and an enlarged spleen. An alternative exploration for these symptoms is the persistence of intestinal worms (Stone 1977). Reiter (2000) demonstrated an elevated mortality rate among children up to 6 years of age living in marshy areas *c.*1800. An innovation in treatment of malaria was the use of cinchona bark. The physician Robert Talbor used this medication *c.*1679 to treat Charles II based on his experiences in Essex (Siegel and Pynter 1962).

Diet made its contribution to the state of health. The Irish were credited with a diet featuring some meat, fish and seafood, wheat and barley loaves, milk and milk products. Potatoes were in use, although the tuber had not yet become the monodiet of the poor (Clarkson and Crawford 2001). Harvests were always at risk due to disease and the weather. In the first half of the seventeenth century Ireland suffered the loss of the harvest in 1601, 1627, and 1648 (Gillespie 1984). Fish were available to some, although the results of commercial fishing were unpredictable; Sir William Petty's plans for large-scale fishing in Kerry were as unprofitable as his iron works there. On the other hand, John Aubrey noted that Edward Davenant "did sett up a fishery … in Ireland where in 20 years he gott 10,000 pounds …" (Dick 1949).

The habitus of people in the seventeenth century can be approximated. Lenihan (1997) put the heights of Irish men and women at 62 and 59 inches, respectively. Then as now teeth were a problem, and the natural philosopher Edmund Halley, of comet fame, lost all his teeth (Allebone 1975).

Stalking all countries was the spectre of bubonic plague; largely an urban disease it like several others was a particular threat to urban immigrants. The disease reached Dublin in 1650 where Sir William Petty estimated the deaths at 275,000 people of all ages. Plague reached London in 1625 and returned in 1665 reaching its peak in September of that year. An account of the plague was given by Samuel Pepys.

> (10 August:) … in great trouble to see the Bill (of Mortality) this week rise so high, to above 4,000 in all, and of them 3,000 of the plague … (31 August.) "the plague having a great increase this week beyond all expectation of almost 2,000, making the general Bill 7,000, odd 100; and the plague above 6,000 … It is feared that the true number of the dead this week is near 10,000.

Of course, Pepys' account covers all ages, but the age pyramid was largely youthful, so that we can infer the death of many children. Landers (1987) reported mortality rates among London's Quakers for the period 1675–1699. Among 577 children ages birth to 9 years I calculate that 45% occurred in the first year of life; 19% of the deaths occurred among children between one and two years for a cumulative 65%. Among the little children ages 2–4 years mortality was 23%, and among the 5–9 year-old group mortality fell to 12% of the recorded deaths. It should be noted that Quakers were not a random group, and it is likely that the general population would have yielded higher percentages at early ages among the deaths acknowledged in the Bills of Mortality.

3.5 Therapy

Given the prevalence of disease and death among the young there arises the matter of what could be done when a child became ill. John Evelyn could send for a doctor, and ordinary people would call for an "empiric" who probably was a quack. At the heart of the matter was the lack of knowledge of disease beyond a grasp of symptoms. The theory of bodily humours prevailed (Arikha 2007) and physicians tended to theorize solutions based on fallacy. Bleeding was a common therapy and probably contributed to mortality rather than to its reduction. One of the few graduates in medicine from Trinity College Dublin was Benjamin Worsley. Called on to prescribe for his friend Robert Boyle his prescription for a malignant fever was, "Apply to the soles of both feet once in twelve hours. Three parts of leaven, one part of Pigeon's dung; & one part of Onyons & Garlicke made up into a kind of Paste with a little Turpentine." Use of snake dung was advised to treat tuberculosis until the dawn of the twentieth century (Smith 1988).

For the seventeenth century parents who chose to develop their own remedies there was a book first published in Latin in 1618. About a half-century late, Nicholas Culpeper translated this work into English thereby enlarging the audience for the work. *Pharmacopeia londinensis of The London Dispensatory* was published by Culpeper in 1654; in it there were treatises on several subjects—*Vide*, "Anatomy of the Body," and "A Treatise of the Ricketts." Culpeper recommended his nostrum, *Aurum Portabile*, which "Cures all agues, whether Quotidian, Tertian, or Quartan, as it also saved diverse people of the most horrid, putrid fever." The book also listed all manner of plants suitable for compounding into remedies, but with the warning, "Let him have a care he mistake not one thing for another. Viz. Herbs for Roots, or either of them for Flowers." The work also included commentaries on the Scriptures.

On the other hand, there was the physician Thomas Arthur (1593–1675) who achieved success and an excellent reputation among the elite of the time in Ireland. In 1656 he treated successfully the tonsillitis experienced by Oliver Cromwell.

Effective physicians commanded high fees, and usually were unavailable to ordinary people. A figure of the times—an era known for its credulity—was Valentine Greatrakes of Waterford. In his heyday Greatrakes appeared before Charles II, and he was patronized by Robert Boyle. In his person "Greatrakes the Stroker," who claimed healing powers in his hands, was a modest, pious man who saw himself as sharing in God's favor. He claimed cures, and others credited him with effective massages (Kaplan 1982). Suggestion probably explained his successes among the more credulous of his clients. In the late 1660s Greatrakes returned to farming in Waterford. Healing hands appear to have been a recognized gift among religious radicals; a prominent man in Dublin's political establishment, Sir Hierome Sankey, claimed that gift had been showered down on him, but without the largesse garnered by Valentine Greatrakes.

3.6 Mortality in Seventeenth Century Dublin

Urban centers provide an opportunity to examine mortality; they present a population of some size, and Dublin was the second city of the British Isles. Like London, Dublin published Bills of Mortality; they were dissected by the analyst of the era, Sir William Petty, who had received the documents from Sir John Temple. Petty noted, "What a shame it is, that these and many other accompts are no better kept" (Lansdowne 1928). Further complicating the situation was the loss, by fire, of public records in 1922. However, Dublin's parishes maintained records which the Parish Register Society made available in the earliest years after 1900.

There are some accounts from the seventeenth century which give a picture of quality of life in Dublin. McLysart (1939) quoted two visitors about life in the city; one called it, "the most pleasant and delightful of the kingdom;" perhaps more realistic was the visitor who said that, "The streets are much pestered with hucksters sitting under bulks whereby the streets are made so narrow that coaches or carts cannot well pass or turn … narrow alleys scarce five feet wide to the danger of ragged children playing in them" (Table 3.2).

It is possible to combine information from various caches of data to shed some light on circumstances affecting child mortality in Dublin's seventeenth century residents. I calculate the proportion of people aged 27 or young at 40% of a group of 495 people in the environs of Dublin (Jordan 2010a–c). The chorography of the city consisted of about 18 parishes—the number varied as parishes were combined (e.g., St. Catherine and St. James) and new ones were added (St. Michans was augmented by he addition of two parishes). To this we can add parish data on hearths—a measure of socio-economic level—births, burials, and availability of piped water (Clark 1987). From these variables comes a scenario which can be summarized as a decided drop in mortality for parishes with access to piped water. Given the persistent threat of disease acquired from contaminated water access to the tiny quantities available to Dublin households and businesses for a fee was a definite asset and probably kept many young children alive. However, primitive pipes could spread water-borne diseases.

3.7 Seventeenth Century London

In 1662, John Graunt, Haberdasher, Officer in the Trained Band, and acquaintance of Oliver Cromwell, published his, *Natural and Political Observation Mentioned in a Following Index, and Made Upon the Bills of Mortality*. This work whose authorship has sometimes been erroneously ascribed to Sir William Petty analyzed 229, 250 deaths dating back to 1623. The Bills were developed, according to Graunt, as follows. "The Searchers … (who are antient Matrons sworn to their Office) … make their report to the Parish-Clerk, and he, every Tuesday night, carries in an Accompt to the Clerk of the Hall. On Wednesday the general Accompt is made up … and on Thursdays published … four shillings per Annum." While numerically accurate, Graunt recognized the weakness of the system in

Table 3.2 Dublin Parishes 1670–1672 and quality of housing by rank

Parish	Housing quality rank	Parish	Housing quality rank
St. Katherine &	12	St. Warburgh (P)	3
St. James (P)[a]		St. Audoen	6
St. Nicholas W'out (P)	8	St. Michael (P)	4
St. Michan	13	St. Keaven	11
St. Andrew with	10	St. Nicholas W'in (P)	2
Donabrook		St. Patrick Liberties	7
St. Bridget	9	Christ Church &	
St. John (P)	5	Trinity College	1

My estimate based on the number of dearths (Butlin 1965)
[a] Access to piped water

terms of nosology. "The old women Searchers after the mist of a cup of Ale, and the bribe of a two-groat fee, instead of one …" might see their way to avoid recording a scandalous cause of death. In some instances conditions we think quite separate were combined, as in "overlaid and starved at nurse."

Despite these considerations Graunt's account of a quarter-million souls sheds light on child deaths across several decades of the seventeenth century. In 1603 there was "the greatest plague-year of this age," a statement which would be overrun 3 years after Graunt's monograph by the great plague of 1665. Among the children lost in 1665 was "an ingeniose youth," son of the talented artist, Wenceslas Hollar, recorded John Aubrey.

In 1632 there were 9,535 deaths recorded in the Bills; the number included 2,268 "Chrysomes and Infants," plus "445 abortive and stillborn." 1632 recorded seven infants whose deaths were set down by the Searchers as "overlaid and starved at nurse." This category combines quite different causes, and it probably under records the numbers. Overlaying was ascribed in later, more critical times to alcoholism, and is, perhaps, an example of a category in which the Searchers made their entries through "the mist of a cup of Ale." In 1659, Bills recorded 226 babies dying in the process of childbirth. One year later, Ricketts was recorded as the cause of death in 521 cases; this nutritional deficiency was combined with "liver-grown, and spleen," conditions we cannot accurately decipher. Graunt gave a picture of early mortality, asserting from his review of just over a quarter-million entries that, "We have found, that of 100 quick Conceptions about thirty six of them die before they be 6 years old." Graunt provided this account of survivorship:

"Viz. of 100 there dies			
Within the first six years	36	The fourth	6
The next ten years, or		The next	4
Decad	24	The next	3
The second decad	15	The next	2
The third decad	09	The next	1

From whence it follows, that of the said 100 conceived there remains alive at six years end 64."

3.8 Eighteenth Century Ireland and England

Data-centered inquiry into the deaths of children in the following century in both England and Ireland is compromised by the relative absence of precise information. For example, smallpox was viewed as a hazard to be faced as a normal expectation for children; but extant data providing dis-aggregation by age are rare. It is evident that deaths from smallpox recorded in the London Bills of Mortality fell across the seventeenth century, but there appears to be only gross analyses by age in early documents (Landers 1987). However, by 1840, Dr. George Gregory could identify two decades beginning in the late eighteenth century, 1797–1817, as a period in which smallpox was relatively absent across western Europe, including the United Kingdom.

3.8.1 England

In 1750, Short published his *New Observations, Natural, Moral, Civil, Political, and Medical, on City, Town, and Country Bills of Mortality*. Short's Table 15 presented numbers from 405,951 deaths between January 1, 1728 and January 1, 1743—a span of 15 years. Table 15 in Short's monograph analyzed deaths in age groups. In the group under 2 years the number of deaths was 148,157, which is 36.62% of the total. The age group "2–5" experienced 14,713 deaths, so that deaths up to and including the fifth birthday amounted to 184,836 babies and little children—which is 45.53% of the total number of deaths. In 1836, Edmonds gave an account of mortality rates for under-fives across the eighteenth century as follows: 1730–1749 = 74.50%; 1750–1769 = 63%; 1770–1789 = 51.50%. Edmonds analyzed mortality in the previous century: "In the 20 years 1730—49, he wrote, out of 100 born, 74.5 died under the age of 5 years." For the northern city of York in the years 1770–1831, the proportion of deaths under 5 years was 36.44% (Laycock 1844).

For adults and children in the eighteenth century Colyton provides mortality data (Wrigley 1968); in Sharpe's (2002) extensive exploration the era 1700–1749 recorded a death rate in Colyton averaging 67.66 per 1,000 children under 5 years of age. For those under one year the rate was 98 per 1,000; for babies between one and 4 years the rate per 1,000 was 82. It then fell sharply among those in the 5–9 years segment at 23 per 1,000. Colyton remains a small community and in the eighteenth century it was infinitely removed from the metropolis. There, the complex of filth and overcrowding created an appalling quality of life which posed the threat of epidemics. Mortality rates recorded in London's Bills of Mortality were higher than those in Colyton to the west, and higher than those in three Yorkshire parishes examined by Levene (2006). In Colyton Sharpe (2002) found a life expectancy of 41.80 years.

Eighteenth century London was a crowded, dirty, overpopulated place astride a filthy Thames—the local sewer—which would not be tackled until the "Great Stink" of 1859. In 1751, William Hogarth advertised "Beer Street and Gin Lane" which conveyed the squalor and drunkenness encountered daily in St. Giles; "Drunk for a penny, dead drunk for twopence" was a familiar enticement. In Hogarth's print, Gin Lane, a drunken woman let her infant fall from her arms to its death. The Bills of Mortality for the middle decades placed mortality for children under five at 44.72% (Pinchbeck and Hewitt 1969). Within this morbid quality of life Captain Thomas Coram (1668–1751) sought to rescue children; in the 1740s Coram established the London Foundling Hospital. It could help only a fraction of London's abandoned children, but its archives provide a window into the lives of children. In Levene's (2005) analysis the years 1756 and 1759 experienced infant mortality rates of 727.7 and 726 per 1,000, the latter for children under one year of age. The Foundling Hospital relied on outplacement of nurslings to the care of wet nurses to age five; survivors were educated to about age 11, and then indentured.

3.8.2 Ireland

In the case of eighteenth century Ireland, we consider a society operating under the penal laws which deprived the *mere Irish*, as they were all too often called, of their civil rights, and which were intended to suppress the majority religion. Across the decades the primary feature was civil unrest, and rural acts of violence. Nature compounded the problems of the eighteenth century; there were three winters, 1728–1730, of "the Bloody Flux" which killed young and old in great numbers, according to Dr. William Wilde (1843). It is not until the end of the eighteenth century that data on circumstances of life, and by implication, of death also, become available (Jordan 2011a, b).

In 1703, the Dublin Workhouse opened and gave shelter to a fraction of the adults and children living on the streets. Originally, children under age five were the responsibility of the local parish, and their care was funded by the *cess*. The survival of foster children was to be protected by quarterly visits, but at SS. Catherine and James the process was reversed; Luke Lowther was required to present his ward to the vestry annually (Gillespie 2004).

In the case of the Workhouse and Foundling Hospital, 4,025 children were admitted in the first 7 years, and their mortality was 80.38%, which is four out of five boys and girls. Between 1737 and 1743 the mortality rate remained high, at about 75%. For the years 1750–1759 the mortality rate rose to 89%, and between 1756 and 1771 the rate fell to about 70% (Robins 1980). Given the funding and arrangement of the facility, the quality of life was little better than life on the streets at best.

In 1798, The Anglican Rector of St. James, a parish large in population and acreage in southwest Dublin, conducted a survey of Dublin's housing (Jordan 2011a, b). The Rev. Mr. Whitelaw's set of 500 tables were not published, but reposed in the Four Courts archives until destroyed by fire in the 1922 civil war. Extant, however, is a brief document which samples Whitelaw's data. From it I calculate that the average population for the 16 parishes south of the river Liffey was 7,031 souls. Whitelaw's parish, St. James, had the largest population—20,176 men, women, and children.

I calculate the density of population at an average of 169 persons per acre, with the most crowding in the parish of St. Michael, where the density was 439 persons per acre. North of the Liffey, the ancient parish of St. Michan was augmented by the establishment of four other parishes. Even so, St. Michan's retained a population of 18,092 persons as the population north of the Liffey expanded.

Whitelaw gave an account of what he and his assistants found when they entered alleyways and crowded tenements:

> A single apartment in one of these truly wretched habitations, rates from one to two shillings per week; and to lighten the rent, two, three, and even four families, become joint tenants. I have frequently surprised from ten to 16 persons, of all ages and sexes, in a room not fifteen feet square, stretched on a wad of filthy straw, swarming with vermin, and without any covering, save the wretched rags that constituted their wearing apparel. In July, 1798, the entire side of a house, four stories high, in School-House Lane, fell from its foundation … the landlord claimed, and received for it, the usual rent … from the thirty persons who had not deserted their apartments.

Given the relatively low rate of improvement in Dublin life across the eighteenth and early nineteenth century it is not unreasonable to apply Short's (1750) eighteenth century estimates of survival to the era of Whitelaw's Dublin. Had the 0–5 years group survived there would have been, in each parish, the number of children given in Table 3.3. The first three columns are taken from the closest reliable account, which is the census of 1821. There is a wide range of population among Dublin's parishes; St. Mary's and St. Michan's had the most residents, while St. Michael's and St. Werburgh's had the smallest populations. There are two parishes named for St. Nicholas; one was within the ancient walls and once was outside.

The third column of numbers, lists by parish, lists the number of children under 5 years who died in 1821, using Short's (1750) incidence of deaths in that age group. Within a total of an estimate of 16,451 deaths the two largest concentration—St. Mary's and St. Michan's—saw over 2,000 deaths of little children. Those numbers are larger than two entire parish populations, St. Michael's and St. Nicholas Within the Walls. The final column in Table 3.3 is an estimate of what parish populations of little children might have been in the absence of the many deaths. The numbers entered there are the sum of the second and third columns of numbers. For example, the first parish in Table 3.3, St. Andrew's, might have had 1,518 living children under age 5 years had not death in many forms intervened.

However, the reality of the era was far different. There was the typhus epidemic of 1817–1819 followed by repeated outbreaks in 1822 and 1826 (O'Neill 1973). This disease was transmitted by the bite of the louse, and is one of the diseases of personal hygiene still encountered by travelers. The year following the census,

Table 3.3 Estimated mortality of children 5 years and under: Dublin 1821

Parishes	Population	Survivors	Died[a]	Potential
St. Andrew's	7,726	903	615	1,518
St. Anne's	8,689	858	584	1,442
St. Audoen's	5,180	638	435	1,072
St. Bridget's	10,36	1,390	947	2,337
St. Catherine's ("Part of")	17,472	2,449	1,668	4,117
St. James's ("Part of")	5,862	678	462	1,140
St. John's	4,408	606	413	1,019
St. Mary's	22,902	2,958	2,015	4,973
Donnybrook ("Part of")	7,278	1,187	808	1,995
St. Michan's	22,92	3,138	2,136	5,276
St. Mark's	11,809	1,628	946	2,828
St. Michael's	1,748	210	143	353
St. Nicholas (W'in)	1,582	221	150	371
St. Nicholas (W'out)	8, 922	1,200	817	2,017
St. Werburgh's	2,620	310	211	521
St. Paul's	12,811	1,623	1,105	2,728
St. Peter's	16,202	1,869	1,273	3,142
St. Thomas's	17,108	2,229	1,518	3,747
Total	185,881	24,149	16,451	40,600

[a] 40.52% mortality (Short 1750)

1822, saw famine return to Ireland, but not on the scale to come in 1846. Facilities to treat sick children were few, although the Dublin Foundling Hospital had been established in 1796. Millin's (1914) account of that institution is informative; over a period of 6 years 12,786 children were admitted, of whom 76.64% died—which is three out of four children.

Our knowledge of children's deaths in the years before the famine years of 1846–1850 comes from the censuses of Ireland conducted in each decade beginning in 1821 (Jordan 1997). Ideally, consideration of death among young children might originate in detailed and sound records, but such is not the case. Dr. William Wilde, physician and father of the playwright, noted that lying-in hospitals kept poor records. In the instance of 2,258 dead infants, "only three causes of death have been assigned, viz, 1 from Syphilis, 4 from convulsions, and 4 from Tetanus. In 2,249 cases … the cause of death has not been stated."

However, inquiries conducted by Dr. Wilde inform our knowledge of the early period. The elder Wilde's *Report Upon the Table of Death*, in 1843, summarized data for the decade 1831–1841.

Apart from the numerical data language indicative of a modernizing frame of mind, the investigation is noteworthy because Dr. Wilde sought to introduce a sense of the social class structure into the data by his characterization of various

Table 3.4 Death: Birth to 15 years, Dublin, by socio-economic level, 1831–1841

Age	1st class private	2nd class private	1st class shop	2nd class shop	3rd class shop	3rd class mixed	Total	%
≤1 Year	124	188	206	906	787	372	2,583	35.53
1–5	152	173	270	1,357	1,145	457	3,554	48.89
6–10	37	42	63	289	230	97	758	10.42
11–15	34	27	27	151	72	62	373	5.13
Total	347	430	566	2,703	2,234	988	7,268	–

sets of streets north and south of the Liffey. In Table 3.4 which is an extract from Wilde's opaque spread sheet (*General Report*, p. lxxv), the presence of retail stores—shops—represents degrees of middle class and lower strata in Dublin society. Some names familiar today identify various streets. First class private streets included Merrion Square, while second class streets may be illustrated by Baggot Street. Shop streets of the first class are represented by Grafton Street. Typically, Wilde named a dozen streets north and south of the Liffey to demonstrate a social gradient in quality of life.

Wilde described a total of twenty-seven districts in Dublin, "… according to their wealth, character, more or less health positions, and the occupations of their populations." It may be noted that Wilde included gender in his data, an element aggregated here; in fact, gender differences in the number of deaths in Wilde's demonstrated more deaths in males.

Table 3.4 shows the greatest percentage of deaths in the third decade of the nineteenth century among the young occurred in the years from 1–5, followed by deaths in the first year, and a decline subsequently. However, when we take into account the number of years the average for each of the years for ages 1–5 declines to 711 per annum. The arithmetic mean is always fictional to a degree, and an average for the 5 years of age is misleading. It is likely that the incidence of deaths would have been highest for the children in the ages 1–2 years group, falling in the remaining 4 years of the quinary. The preponderance of deaths occurred in the second and third class streets. Wilde's data set is important because it demonstrated to the Victorians that the social aspect of mortality was inseparable from the quality of life. The poor died in large numbers at all ages, and their little children were no exception in the Liberties and similar concentrations of the poor.

In 1833 Commissioners were appointed to inquire "… Into the Condition of the Poorer Classes in Ireland" (1835). In County Carlow, the Grand Jury noted the risk to life among illegitimate infants. Lieutenant Battersby, the Chief Constable, said that,

> there are 50 illegitimate children and foundling children in this parish (Carlow parish), 10 of whom are supported by it. Mothers frequently desert their children. There is a woman at present in gaol for the offence, who was offered her liberty if she would take the child, and refused. They frequently destroy them. Lieutenant Battersby, J. P. states that he held three inquests within the last 14 months on destroyed children … They are sometimes found floating in the river.

3.8.3 Famine

However, the appalling rate of mortality in the 1830s would soon be exceeded by the effects of the infestation of the potato crop by the organism, *Phytophthera infestans Mont.* Recalling that nineteenth century Ireland was a rural country for the most part, underlines the role of a relatively cash-free economy when the major crop fails. Famine in Victorian Ireland did not mean that there was no food; in fact, Ireland exported food products. Those with cash could find food, but not the potato which had evolved into a monodiet for the rural poor. The deaths of adults and children came about from starvation, in many cases, but the intercurrent cause was communicable disease as starvation ravaged the immune system. In 1851 there was another census, and Dr. Wilde was an Under Commissioner. In the *General Report* for 1851 (1856), Table XXXIII listed annual deaths by town and province. In 1846, the number of deaths across Ireland's 32 counties and four provinces was 122, 889; it then expanded across the years and declined sharply in 1850: 1847 = 249,335, 1848 = 208,252, 1849 = 240,797, 1850 = 164,093. Interacting with disease in the number of deaths was the phenomenon of emigration, both voluntary and involuntary, as landlords cleared their acres. In 1841, the census Commissioners had counted 8,175,124 persons—a number which had shrunk to 6,552,385 in 1851.

Amidst this carnage the prior number of child deaths is not discernible in the 1851 census data. For the years 1847–1850 the total number of deaths was 862,477 persons. However, Grada (1988) put the number of deaths among 4-year olds at 285,000, and among children under 9 years at 472,000. Circumstances in those years combined predictable deaths in ordinary times with those due to malnutrition and disease.

The workhouse at Navan saw the death in 1848 of Anne Monaghan, age six; 38 other children under 8 years also died. In the case of Bridget and James Early, ages 5 and 4 years, death came through the mechanism of diarrhea and dysentery (Connell 2004). Three estimates of the child component of all deaths in the 5-year period are: 5% = 34,129; 10% = 86,247; and 15% = 129,371. Within those numerical estimates are variations due to place and local outbreaks of particular diseases, and the vulnerability of infants at the best of times.

However, fate had not finished with Ireland; in 1849 cholera appeared. Here too death was a matter of hygiene, the *vibrio* was transmitted easily and swiftly from person to person at a time when human waste was frequently encountered in the home and neighborhood. Once stricken the victim did not linger, and death by dehydration could occur in less than 12 h. The children who did not die in the famine years or in the years after cholera were not without after effects; reports from the era indicate extensive presence of physical, mental, and emotional consequences.

On the Sister Island to Ireland, as the Victorians euphemistically named both of the British Isles, the processes of change affected childhood more radically. Landers' (1987) analysis of deaths in London covered the years 1680–1819. Over those 140 years the percentage of deaths in "infancy" rose from 28.20 in the decade 1680–1689 to 39.90% in the decade 1730–1739; the rate of such deaths then fell steadily, and the last decade, 1810–1819, recorded a rate of 29.80%.

At the end of the eighteenth century the Industrial Revolution began in the form of factories powered by steam—but also by the labor of little children. Relevant, but beyond the scope of this essay, are accounts of the appalling working conditions in factories and mines to which small children were exposed (Chadwick 1842; Jordan 1987a, b, 1993a, b). In relation to the death of children, the causes of mortality included the epidemical diseases of childhood, plus the recurrent waves of exceptional diseases such as cholera which arrived from the continent in 1832, 1848, 1854, and for the last time, in 1866. Cholera was traced by "The Great Chadwick" (1844a, b) to "bad water, bad air, defective drainage, overcrowding, dirty and irregular habits;" he also pointed out that cholera was transmitted by one infected person to one or more other persons.

In Table 3.5 are annual data from Mitchell and Deane on deaths of children under 2 years presented here in units of five calendar years for England and Wales, and Ireland in the years 1838–1902, the years for Ireland beginning later, in 1863. The symbols *H* and *L* identify the highest and lowest annual rates in the series.

In all years across the Victorian era the rates reported from Ireland were below those for England and Wales (as were rates from Scotland which resembled Ireland more than England and Wales). The 13 quinquennial rates in Table 3.5 decline and rise across the span of 64 years around a mean rate 150.60 deaths of children under 2 years per year; representative is the 5-year period, 1858–1862. In the case of the "sister island," the mean rate for the briefer series of eight quinaries is 98.04, and the rate of 97.20 in 1888–1892 is typical. For both islands comparison shows that the rate in England and Wales was about half again as much as in Ireland. On both islands the annual mortality for little children in the Victorian era changed little, and is appalling by modern standards.

3.9 Cultural Factors

Victorian Britain and Ireland facilitate consideration of some causes of early child mortality which are more qualitative than numerical. They are elements of the culture of Victorian society which predisposed children toward a brief life.

3.9.1 Ireland

In 1641 Sir Phelim O'Neill began an unsuccessful uprising against British rule. The result was a decade of violence and death leading up to Oliver Cromwell's swift and effective campaign in 1649. In the decade of the 1640s Irish people died

Table 3.5 Mortality among Children <2 years, England and Wales, and Ireland, 1838–1902

Year	England and Wales	Ireland
1838–1842	150.50	–
1843–1847	153.60	–
1848–1852	157.20 *H*	–
1853–1857	153.00	–
1858–1862	149.40	–
1863–1867	155.00	96.75
1868–1872	155.80	94.20 *L*
1873–1877	148.00	94.20 *L*
1878–1882	142.20 *L*	94.20
1883–1887	143.20	94.80
1888–1892	145.60	97.20
1893–1897	152.20	102.40
1898–1802	152.20	105.60 *H*
1838–1902	$M = 150.60$	$M = 98.40$
1863–1902	$M = 149.20$	$M = 92.40$

Mitchell and Deane (1971)

in huge numbers (Lenihan 1997). In close succession came plague which, according to Sir William Petty, physician and empiricist, carried off 412,500 people across Ireland.

In later years, capped by the failure of the potato crop in the late 1840s, Irish children's prospects for a long life were at risk due to appalling living conditions. A rural people, the Irish lived—or existed—in hovels. Through their abodes ran chickens and pigs ("The Gintleman that pays the rint"), and the smoke of a peat fire floated around and then drifted through a hole in the roof. There were no amenities and material poverty was acute. Dwellings were usually little more than an unreliable defence against the elements. In such settings infants and little children were exposed to frequent infections. Scarlet fever and smallpox were hazards for children to face routinely; scarlet fever was then a near-fatal disease.

3.9.2 England and Wales

Across the centuries the population steadily became urbanized, a process speeded up by the Industrial Revolution. In the increasingly dense urban context of the factory towns communicable diseases spread rapidly, and family life deteriorated.

3.9.3 Godfrey's Cordial

Fussy children and those with more serious problems needed soothing; available at the local pharmacy or from the "crocus" man who went door to door was Godfrey's Cordial. The opium derivative, laudanum, was the basis for this often fatal opiate. Indeed, it amounted to the sovereign remedy when a nurse needed to sedate a child. In some instances the cordial was given almost automatically at birth to newborns (Jordan 1987b). This medication was not prescribed by physicians, but midwives and other attendants had ready access to the fatal soporific. In eighteenth century Dublin this opiate was known as *diacodium* (Robins 1980). At the highest levels of public affairs in Victorian Britain Dr. William Farr (1868) warned that "a few drops of laudanum are fatal" to the newborn. A few years before, the Ladies Sanitary Association (1860) embarked on a program to educate mothers in rudimentary practices for a healthy family life. Little poems were aimed at ignorant mothers about the dangers of common medicines:

> Don't give him sleeping draughts
> to hurt his tender brain,
> But keep him clean, and fresh, and cool,
> To soothe the heat and pain.

3.9.4 Baby Farming

Not every birth was welcome in nineteenth century Britain, and there evolved a form of infanticide with a disarming name. An illegitimate or otherwise inconvenient baby could be silently and effectively removed from the scene. One merely looked in the newspaper for a discretely worded advertisement offering to adopt or to relieve interested parties of infants to be boarded out for a fee. In one scenario procurers posed as a couple seeking to adopt a child. The Rev. Benjamin Waugh (1890) recalled conversations with "farmers"—"Talk of syrups and laudanum, and they will cautiously smile assent;" he added that, "It is as easy to get a baby's life out of it as it is to rub the dust from a butterfly's wing." (for anecdotes about baby farming see Waugh 1890; Pinchbeck and Hewitt 1973). In a curious turn of phrase in H.M.S. Pinafore, Little Buttercup acknowledges that she had taken up baby farming, "… when I was young and charming, many years ago."

3.9.5 Climbing Boys

The abundance of coal fires left the winter atmosphere in towns a dark cloudy miasma. Most of the energy went up the chimney as smoke, while a modicum heated the room. Routinely, chimneys caught fire, and the remedy was to sweep the chimney in advance. To do so required brushes, but small boys fitted chimneys quite well, and could be directed from the fireplace. Boys as young as five and six were recruited into this dangerous trade from the ranks of the poor and abandoned. (Chimneys and Chimney sweepers 1844). The smaller (i.e., younger) the boy the better to climb and sweep chimneys from within. The hazards were the accumulated soot which the boys ingested, the risk of falling, and the long-term risk of cancer—Pott's disease—a form of cancer unique to chimney sweeps. The end of the practice did not come easily; there were home owners who insisted that brushes were not good enough, and that the risk of fire in a chimney required the use of climbing boys.

3.9.6 Industrialization

The price for industrialization was evident in the towns of England and Scotland. In the early decades the unhinging of small town and village life led to social anomie and the abuse of children. Factory work by little children endangered them in two ways. There was the risk posed by working amidst machinery, but there was the more obvious assault by supervisors who used physical punishment to discipline child workers. At age seven Robert Blincoe was sent from the St. Pancras workhouse in London to labor in a Lancashire cotton mill about 200 miles to the north. In his adult years Robert Blincoe was described as "a little man in height, his legs being very crooked, the result of his early life in a cotton factory … one Richard Goodall, he describes as entirely beaten to death." (Browne 1832).

Less visible was the risk to life and limb posed to little children by working underground in mines. In an era when only candle light was available, small children pulled carts of coal along tracks far under ground. In an 1842 report the Children's Employment Commission noted that, "Many of the infants in a collier (mine) community are thin, skinny, and wasted, and indicate by their constricted features and sickly dirty white or faintly yellowish aspect their early participation in a deteriorated physical condition. The physical condition of the boys and girls engaged in the collieries is much inferior to that of children of the same years … in most trades …"

At the end of the nineteenth century the Manchester district, Angel Meadow, was described by the Rev. Mercer (1897). In an area of about 23 acres over 7,000 people reside; that density converts to 212.12 persons per acre. Under such conditions the childhood diseases flourished bringing sickness and death to all segments of the population, but especially to the youngest. After providing statistics on the overcrowding and unsanitary conditions Mercer (1897) recalled that, "Not long ago I found the mother of a family lying dead, the younger children playing round the bed and turning up the sheets in curiosity to examine the body, and the elder girl washing up on a table near the bed, and leaning the pots against the mother's legs to drain."

Table 3.6 Child mortality <10 years by occupational group ($N = 1{,}779$)

Parental occupation	% died	% Epidemic deaths	Mean age at death all subjects
Gentlemen	28	4	45
Farmers & c	18	7	47
Labourers	28	10	39
Paupers	30	4	5
Undescribed	53	15	30

Chadwick (1844a, b)

From a variety of social malfunctions and a sense of impending doom the Victorians began to assemble data on the health of the nation. A series of commentaries drew the conclusion that the British people had entered a decline in their overall health which was progressive, and probably irreversible (Jordan 1993a, b). This last element interacted with the prevailing misconceptions of genetics, and led to public inquiries. In time, legislation would improve the health of children and so reduce their risk of an early death due to communicable disease and filth. However, Victorian Britain was burdened by a caste system in which socio-occupational status influenced rates of mortality even in places far removed from urban squalor. Table 3.6 presents a reanalysis of data from 1839 aggregated by Chadwick (1844a, b) from the bucolic county of Herefordshire.

The percentage of children under 10 years dying in Herefordshire increases in Table 3.6 as the occupational status declines; on the other hand, the percentage of deaths due to epidemical diseases rises. Finally, to project the lifelong significance of class membership beyond 10 years, it is apparent in Table 3.6 that the anomic "Undescribed" at the bottom of the social hierarchy died well before their more favored brethren.

It took about six decades to move from Edwin Chadwick's reports in the 1840s to the awakening sense that reforming legislation could raise the quality of life. Even so, heights appear to have remained low by today's standards until after the 1914–1918 war. A corollary was the high rate of rejection among young men volunteering to serve Queen and Country (Jordan 1993a, b).

3.10 Date and Perspective

Objectivity in the matter of death among children takes two forms; there is the objectivity of numerical formulations which is intended to yield rational appraisals. A second form is a degree of emotional detachment from a painful state of mind. This chapter has sought to use the former, while the latter has been aided by the distance in time and from the era under consideration. To a degree, detachment has been attributed to parents for whom the death of children, one's own or those of relatives and friends, was an all too common experience. Pinchbeck and Hewitt (1969) discussed the bereavement experience by parents, and quoted an appraisal of Samuel Johnson's friend, Mrs. Hester Thrale, as showing "great equanimity" regarding "the deaths of various daughters at a school." Sir John Verney lost two of his 15 children, and was said to have observed that he still had a baker's dozen.

That such equanimity was widespread in view of the frequency of children's deaths can be both facile and misleading. John Evelyn's frame of mind may be inferred from his diary entry for 27 January 1658. Regarding the death of 5 year old Dick, Evelyn recorded: "He would of himselfe select the most pathetic psalms, and chapters out of Job, to reade to his mayde during his sickness, telling her when she pitied him that all God's children much suffer affliction ... Such a child I never saw; for such a child I blesse God in whose bosome he now is ! ... Here ends the joy of my life, and for which I go even mourning to the grave."

Toward the end of the next century, in April 1796, Elizabeth Dean, aged 5 years and nine months, died and was interred in the crypt at St. Martin in the Fields. It seems likely that this all too common event moved the emotions of the Dean family deeply.

In the nineteenth century, The Rev. Mr. Patrick Bronte witnessed the sequential deaths from tuberculosis of his talented children. The scientist Thomas Huxley recorded that, "... our Noel, our first-borne, after being for four years our delight and our joy, was carried off by scarlet fever in 48 hours" (Irvine 1959).

In these examples of deep feeling of parents in the face of a tragedy there is the experience of loss several years after birth. Another form of loss is the birth of a still-born infant. An anonymous Victorian mother, "On Visiting the Grave of my Stillborn Little Girl," wrote in 1836:

I made a vow within my soul, O child,
When thou wert laid beside my weary heart,
With marks of Death on every tender part,
That, if in time a living infant smiled,
Winning my ear with gentle sounds of love
In sunshine of such joy, I still would save
A green rest for they memory, O Dove !

In the end the death of children, whether in the seventeenth or twenty-first century, becomes a matter of perspective; that is, there is the continuum of subjective to objective appraisals, and there is the mind and heart polarity of bereaved parent and statistical analyst. By considering both elements the death of children can be appraised as the harsh reality it presents.

When early mortality is considered within a cohort it appears that those who died present implications for the survivors. That is, survivors in a cohort with excessive deaths before age 5 years incur the risk of reduced life expectancies as they age. The survivors in such a cohort tend to die before their predicted life expectancy in a statistically derived process called "diminished entelechy" (Catalano and Bruckner 2006). A corollary would be that reduced early mortality would be beneficial to the cohort in the adult years. That proposition is confounded to a degree by social innovations affecting cohort survivors in later years; e.g., advances in medicine and social policy.

In this consideration of the death of young children the time perspective reveals a change in values of at least two kinds; there is the infusion of number as the data language of inquiry which installed the modernity evident in censuses. It stands in contrast to the prose and poetry of the seventeenth century, so that it seems unlikely that anyone today would express the sentiments expressed by a bereaved father in the seventeenth century (Dick 1949):

> Christopher Michell's son lyeth here, Richard Mitchell was his Name,
> His father's Love was so to him, he caus'd to write the same:
> He was but 4 Years 5 Months old, and then was buryed here,
> And of his Body the Worms did find a Dish of dainty here.

In this verse we see seventeenth century melancholy verbalized as the inevitable corruption of the body, a trope painful but apparently conventional in a century of plagues. This rough verse taken from a tombstone conveys more than a father's loss; it provides a clue to how the death of little children has been received across the centuries. That is, their deaths as recorded here in verse express a set of values which evolve with time. Sometimes described broadly as a world-outlook (*Weltanschaung*), the concept was refined by Maruyama (1980) into Mindscapes, patterns of mental organization, which describe modes of perceiving the world around us. Thus, the death of little children over three centuries has been contained in each era's mindscape. The expression of those deaths, exemplified here in personal reflections, rhyme, and statistics, reveals the social construction of the deaths of little children, an event once commonplace but now exceptional in the westernized world.

References

Allebone, E. (1975). Edmond Halley and the clubs of the Royal Society. *Notes and Records of the Royal Society of London, 28*, 198–205.

Aries, P. (1962). *Centuries of childhood: A social history of family life*. New York: Vintage.

Arikha, N. (2007). *Passions and tempers: A history of the humours*. New York: Ecco/HarperCollins.

Berry, H. F. (1907). The Registers of the Church of St. Michan, Dublin, 1636–1685. Dublin. Parish Register Society of Dublin.

Berry, H. F. (1909). Registers of the church of St. Michan, Dublin, (Part Two), 1686–1700. Dublin: Parish Register Society of Dublin.

Browne, J. (1832). *A memoir of robert blincoe*. Doherty: Manchester.

Butlin, R. A. (1965). The population of Dublin and the late seventeenth century. *Irish Geography, 5*, 51–66.

Catalano, R., & Bruckner, T. (2006). Child mortality and cohort lifespan: A test of diminishing entelechy. *International Journal of Epidemiology, 35*, 1264–1269.

Chadwick, E. (1842). Report on the sanitary condition of the laboring population of Great Britain. *Parliamentary Papers, 3*, 1–457.

Chadwick, E. (1844a). On the best modes of representing accurately, by statistical returns, the duration of life, and the pressure and progress of the causes of mortality amongst the populations of different districts and countries. *Quarterly Journal of the Statistical Society of London, 7*, 1–40.

Chadwick, E. (1844b). Report on the sanitary condition of the laboring population of Great Britain. *Parliamentary Papers, 3*, 1–457.

Chimneys and chimney sweepers. (1844). *The Penny Magazine*, 322.

Clark, M. (1987). Dublin city piped water accounts. *Irish Genealogist, 7*, 201–204.

Clarkson, L. M., & Crawford, M. (2001). *Feast and Famine: Food and nutrition in Ireland, 1500–1920*. Oxford: Oxford University Press.

Coffman, A. (2009). *"To the memory of sweet infants": Eighteenth century commemorations of child death in tidewater*. Blacksburg: Virginia. M.A. thesis. Virginia Polytechnic and State University.

Connell, P. (2004). *The land and the people of County Meath, 1750–1850*. Four Courts: Dublin.

Dick, D. L. (1949). *Aubrey's Brief Lives*. Ann Arbor, MI. Ann Arbor Books.

Edmonds, T. R. (1836). Mortality of infants in England. *Lancet*. 690–693.

Farr, W. (1868). Mortality of children in the principal states of Europe. *Journal of the Royal Statistical Society, 29*, 1–35.

First Report from His Majesty's Commissioners for Inquiring into the Condition of the Poorer Classes in Ireland. (1835). *Appendix (A)*. London: House of Commons.

Forbes, T. R. (1974). The searchers. *Bulletin of the New York Academy of Science, 50*, 1031–1038.

Gillespie, R. (1984). Harvest crises in early seventeenth century Ireland. *Irish Economic and Social History, 11*, 5–18.

Gillespie, R. (2004). *The vestry records of the parishes of St. Catherine and St. James, Dublin*. Dublin: Four Courts.

Hawking, S. (2002). *On the shoulders of giants: The great works of physics and astronomy*. Philadelphia: Running Press.

Hill, C. (1975). *The world turned upside down*. London: Pelican.

Irvine, W. (1959). Apes, Angels, and Victorians: Darwin, Huxley, and Evolution. Cleveland, OH. World.

Jardine, L., & Silverthorne, M. (2000). *Francis bacon: The new organon*. Cambridge: Cambridge University Press.

Jordan, T. E. (1987a). *Victorian childhood: Themes and variations*. Albany: State University of New York Press.

Jordan, T. E. (1987b). "The keys of paradise": Godfrey's cordial and children in Victorian Britain. *Journal of the Royal Society of Health, 107*, 19–22.

Jordan, T. E. (1993a). "L'Homme Moyen": Estimating the quality of life for British adults 1815–1914, an index. *Social Indicators Research, 29*, 183–203.

Jordan, T. E. (1993b). *The degeneracy crisis and Victorian youth*. Albany: State University of New York Press.

Jordan, T. E. (1997). A century of Irish censuses. *New Hibernia Review, 2*, 94–114.

Jordan, T. E. (2007). *"A copper farthing": Sir William Petty and his times*. Sunderland: University of Sunderland Press.

Jordan, T. E. (2010a). Quality of family life and mortality in seventeenth century Dublin. *Social Indicators Research, 98*, 251–263.

Jordan, T. E. (2010b). Quality of living conditions in eighteenth century Dublin: Whitelaw's survey, 1798. In, *Studies in the Quality of Life and Human Development in Ireland and Britain Since the Sixteenth Century*. Lewiston, New York: Mellen.

Jordan, T. E. (2010c). *Studies in the quality of life and human development in Ireland and Britain since the sixteenth century*. Lewiston: Mellen.

Jordan, T. E. (2011a). Whitelaw's essay on the population of Dublin (1805): A window on eighteenth century housing. *New Hibernia Review, 15*, 9–18.

Jordan, T. E. (2011b). Whitelaw's essay on the population of Dublin (1805): A window on late eighteenth century housing. *New Hibernia Review, 25*, 136–145.

Kaplan, B. (1982). Greatrakes the stroker: The interpretation of his contemporaries. *Isis, 73*, 178–185.

Kunitz, S. J. (1984). Mortality changes in America, 1620–1920. *Human Biology, 56*, 559–582.

Landers, J. (1987). Mortality and metropolis: The case of London 1675–1825. *Population Studies, 41*, 59–76.

Lansdowne, (1928). *The petty-southwell correspondence 1676–1687*. London: Constable.

Laycock, T. R. (1844). The city of York. Health of Towns Commission. *Parliamentary Papers*, 1844.

Le Gallienne, R. (2003). *The diary of samuel pepys*. New York: Modern Library.

Lenihan, P. (1997). War and population, 1649–1652. *Irish Economic and Social History, 24*, 1–21.

Levene, A. (2005). The estimation of mortality at the London foundling hospital, 1741–99. *Population Studies, 59*, 89–99.

Levene, A. (2006). What can dade registers tell us about infant mortality in later eighteenth century? *Local Population Studies, 76*, 31–42.

Lewis, J. (1998). "Tis a misfortune to be a Great Ladie"; maternal mortality in the British aristocracy, 1588–1959. *Journal of British Studies, 37*, 26–53.

Maruyama, M. (1980). Mindscapes and science theories. *Current Anthropology, 21*, 589–599.

McLysaght, E. (1939). *Irish life in the seventeenth century*. Cork: Cork University Press.

Mercer, J. E. (1897). The condition of life in Angel Meadow. *Transactions of the Manchester Statistical Society*. 158–180.

Millin, S. (1914). A sociological retrospect of Dulin. *Journal of the Statistical and Social Inquiry Society of Ireland, 13*, 130–159.

Mills, J. (1906). *The Registers of St. John the Evangelist, Dublin, 1619–1699*. Dublin: The Parish Registers Society of Dublin.

Mitchell, B. R. (1971). *British historical statistics*. Cambridge: Cambridge University Press.

Morgan, V. M. (1974). Mortality in magherafelt, county derry, in the early eighteenth century. *Irish Historical Studies, 19*, 125–135.

Mullett, C. F. (1938). Sir William Petty on the plague. *Isis, 28*, 18–25.

O Grada, C. (1988). *"For irishmen to forget?": Recent research on the great Irish famine*. Dublin: University College.

O'Neill, T. P. (1973). Fever and public health in pre-famine Ireland. *Journal of the Royal Society of Antiquaries of Ireland, 103*, 1–34.

Petty, W. (1691). *The Political Anatomy of Ireland*. London. Pardoe.

Pinchbeck, I., & Hewitt, M. (1969). *Children in english society. volume i. from tudor times to the eighteenth century* (Vol. I). London: Routledge and Kegan Paul.

Pinchbeck, I., & Hewitt, M. (1973). *Childhood in english society* (Vol. Vols I and II). London: Routledge and Kegan Paul.

Reiter, P. (2000). From shakespeare to defoe: Malaria in England in the little ice age. *Emerging Infectious Diseases, 6*, 1–11.

Robins, J. (1980). *The lost children: charity children in Ireland, 1700–1900*. Dublin: Institute of Public Administration.

Sharpe, P. (2002). *Population and society in an East Devon parish: Reproducing colyton 1540–1640*. Exeter: University of Exetor Press.

Short, T. (1750). *New observations natural, moral, civil, political, and medical on city, town and country bills of mortality*. London: Longman and Millar.

Siegel, R. E., & Pynter, F. N. L. (1962). Robert Tabor, Charles II, and Cinchona: A contemporary document. *Medical History, 6*, 82–85.

Smith, D. B. (1980). *Inside the great house: Planter family life in eighteenth century planter society*. Ithaca: Cornell University Press.

Smith, F. B. (1988). *The retreat of Tuberculosis, 1850–1950*. London: Croom Helm.

Stone, L. (1977). *The family, sex, and marriage in England, 1500–1800*. New York: Harper and Row.

Thrower, N. J. W. (2003). Samuel Pepys F. R. S. (1633–1703) and the Royal Society. *Notes and Records of the Royal Society of London, 57*, 3–13.

Waugh, B. (1890). Baby farming. Contemporary. *Review, 57*, 700–714.

Wilde, W. R. (1843). Report on the Table of Deaths. *Report of the Commissioners Appointed to Take the Census of Ireland, for the Year 1841*. Dublin. Thom.

Wrigley, E. A. (1968). Mortality in pre-industrial England: The example of Colyton, Devon, over three centuries. *Daedalus, 97*, 546–580.

Chapter 4
Children's Mortality in England and Wales: 1838–1902

4.1 Introduction

When William IV's 7-year reign ended in 1837, he had fathered 11 children in an era when death was a frequent occurrence. William left no legitimate heir, his surviving offspring had been born to the Dublin-born actress, Mrs. Dorothea Jordan, with whom he lived in domestic tranquility for two decades. William IV experienced the death of a son, and of two little girls born to his legal spouse, the Princess Adelaide. In that era the death of children was all too familiar to families, but society's emerging modernism had not yet grasped that mortality was a topic related to the formation of public policy, except in a general way when governments reacted to health crises or needed to raise armies. By the middle decade of the nineteenth century, most European countries gathered vital statistics on their populations, and as a result the demography of England and Wales is generally understood (Woods 2000).

In the years encompassed by Queen Victoria's reign, health and social statistics became tools for formation of public policy. The mortality of children was recorded and analyzed, as was the mortality of older age groups. A major finding was the alarming number of working class people whose health was inferior to that of previous generations—the degeneracy crisis (Jordan 1993b).

The Victorian era was dynamic; at its core was the economy which, by 1838, had matured from its origins three decades earlier. Deposits of coal and iron were fairly accessible, and South Wales and the Northeast became centers of production. Evolution of engineering skills led to fabrication of iron bridges and rail lines, and they connected the centers of trade and population. A consequence was the decline of the lengthy system of canals whose capacity and pace were overshadowed by railways. Traffic on canals did not disappear, and families carried on their trade living on their long, narrow boats pulled by horses. Little children played their part, sometimes guiding the beast along the path at the side of the canal. The reformer George Smith called attention to the risk to life and health experienced by

T. E. Jordan, *Quality of Life and Mortality Among Children*,
SpringerBriefs in Well-Being and Quality of Life Research,
DOI: 10.1007/978-94-007-4390-8_4, © The Author(s) 2012

little children in the 1870s. As late as the 1920s, the plight of canal boat children persisted; their mobility left them the responsibility of no one for very long.

Across the nineteenth century commodity prices declined (Kondratieff 1926), and incomes and prices also rose, one canceling the other from time to time. Child mortality slowly declined, but tuberculosis remained a scourge, its source remaining obscure until 1880. A social phenomenon of the nineteenth century was the effort of working men to unionize, and so raise their incomes. Progress came slowly, and children sometimes suffered when families' resources were diverted to ensure the strength of the breadwinner.

Commentators pointed to the paradox of the nation's increasing wealth and expanding empire, while the urban young appeared to be getting weaker with each generation. Rural families were not exempt from the social trends of the era, and there were changes in the diet of farm laborers' families across the last half of the century. Sugar increased in the diet, and skimmed milk—an item quite insufficient for infants—became a regular element in the dietary based on price (Fussell 1929).

The subject of this chapter, mortality among children in the nineteenth century, should be viewed as a correlate of rapid social change. Mature members of Princess Victoria's household could recall the influx of French aristocrats fleeing the tumbrels and guillotine of the revolution; to them the threat of Bonapartism had been real. Ordinary people recalled the economic downturn, when the French threat collapsed with the exile of Napoleon to St. Helena. At the end of the Victorian era, gas light and steam power were overtaken by the telephone, electricity, and the promise of the internal combustion engine. Britain's attachment to coal as an energy source had a persuasive rationale, but it became a hindrance as nations competed in a world economy.

Despite selective advances in aspects of national life, children's health and mortality remained threatened across the decades. A particular exception to progress was the state of medicine; in that field innovations were few; vaccination became common, and in 1880 Dr. Lawson Tait introduced the appendectomy; auxiliary to medical science were the innovations of Florence Nightingale in nursing. The great killer of the age, pulmonary tuberculosis, continued its silent rampage among young and old. The array of change and stability illustrates differential rates of social change in a dynamic society.

As we approach the numerical data of this chapter, it may be recalled that the death of children has an arbitrary aspect. Here, enumeration is at the level of two regions, Victorian England and Wales, and in these principalities there was an incomplete style of gathering information. That is, child mortality data accrued with little recording of social classes and cultural elements, such as poverty (Reid 1977). Urban expansion of this last item is exemplified in Henry Mayhew's (1851) *London Labour and the London Poor* (Quennell 1969).

In recent years, mortality has been differentiated by social and geographic factors (Reid 1997). Lee's (1991) econometric analysis of 55 regions of England, Wales, and Scotland began with mortality rates in 1861; his regression analyzes for 1871 yielded a statistically significant account of criterion variance ($R^2 = 0.24$). The counties employed ranged widely, in that year, in infant mortality per 1,000 live births; from 112 deaths in rural Dorset in the southwest to 186 in industrialized Lancashire in the Northwest. A major influence was the pattern of occupations; heavy industry and mining influenced regions toward higher rates of infant mortality. Families caught up in the migration to industrialized settings had little to support them when there were economic reverses. The Old Poor Law which emphasized local decision-making had limited resources, and could be strict. However, the Old Poor Law now seems to have become, in retrospect, a system with some virtues (Kelly and Grada 2011), in light of the strict requirements of the revised version in 1834, which ended outdoor relief (Crowther 1981).

In the case of the 0–5 age group, England and Wales had neither the best nor the worst survival rates for their youngest. Norway had the lowest early mortality rates—11%, according to data assembled by one of the great figures in Victorian public health, Dr. William Farr (1866). Study of children's mortality in England and Wales in the Victorian era considers a country at extreme for risk to life, and also a prime site to examine mortality within a population experiencing industrialization and the high price that entailed. The mortality of young children amounted to the canary in the coal mine, warning of perilous times.

However, to the population of the United Kingdom the accession of Princess Victoria to the throne vacated by her uncle, William IV, in 1837 was an occasion for optimism. The legacy of the little-known but influential thinker, Jeremy Bentham (1748–1832), had begun an era of progressive utilitarianism. Evolution in the public philosophy was evident in the use of parliamentary inquiries exposing facts. That theme was expressed by Charles Dickens in the person of the character in *Hard Times*, Thomas Gradgrind. However, promising the prospects for quality of life unfolding in steam power, factories, and reforming laws, there were realities which disquieted thoughtful men. Not the least was the declining health of the population of the rising factory towns in the Midlands and northern counties. An accelerating degeneracy crisis seemed at hand (Jordan 1993a, b).

Addressing the Royal Institution in 1840, the Physician to the Smallpox Hospital, Dr. George Gregory, supported his remarks with facts gleaned since the start of registration of births and deaths (but not stillbirths) in 1837. Gregory noted that in manufacturing districts "… one half of those born do not attain the age of 12 years," and that "one half of the males were dead at seven, half the females at seventeen." He was responsive to the influence of environment noting that in the West Riding of Yorkshire, a manufacturing district, "half of those born are gone at 18," but in the agricultural North Riding, "the half are not dead till 38."

4.2 Health and Living Conditions

Across the nineteenth century, mortality was seen as a phenomenon with well-defined correlates. In 1849, Dr. John Snow removed the handle from the Broad Street pump incentral London and reduced the cholera outbreak. However, in an age which relied on the theory of disease due to miasma—poisonous vapors—there were skeptics. Even the great health reformer Dr. John Simon, resisted the *vibrio* source for a decade.

The Victorian mindset sifted as well as gathered facts, and the censuses at intervals of a decade, formalized the idiom of inquiry, glimpsed first as the century had opened. In 1805, James Whitelaw published his survey of the streets and residents of Dublin, then the second city of the British Isles (Jordan 2011a, b). That pioneering work was followed by similar studies undertaken by local statistical societies. Two decades after Whitelaw's inquiries Edwin Chadwick (1828) described working class people criticizing the, "… tyrannical control of (their) appetites and possessions … that propensity to seize with avidity and to use without restraint, the means of immediate gratification." In 1833, James Kay surveyed Manchester cotton workers living in Deansgate—known locally as Devilsgate—among whom he found sickness, dependence on alcohol, and an indifference to religion. In 1838, James Heywood surveyed 999 residents of the nearby Miles Platting district. Heywood (1839) did not like what he unearthed, finding the heads of households, "either too illiterate, or too deeply sunk in indifference, or in animal gratification …" to better themselves or to care for their children. Much the same impression came from the more influential account of the lives of workers given by Friedrich Engels (1845). Clearly, Victorian reformers viewed their clients warily. The way of life of the poor was far removed from that of their advocates; the latter embraced a degree of modernism, a set of values set forth by the writer Samuel Smiles (1880) who called for thrift, delayed gratification, and sobriety.

Not the least victims were the children; the reformer Michael Sadler (Sadler 1833) received an account of a child worker from his fellow advocate, Dr. J. H. Green:

> David Harley is a shocking spectacle, being crippled in both knees, and crooked in both legs. He was sent to the factory at 7 years of age, and very soon began to complain of pain in the ankle and knee joints; and being unable to support himself in an erect position, he used to lean against the frame, with one knee in a bent position, alternately changing them, until he became most shockingly deformed, and irreparably crippled. This poor boy is an illegitimate child, entirely deserted by both father and mother, and is still compelled to work in the factory, or starve; but he is unable to stand upon his feet, and is obliged to kneel at his work from morning to night.

Even at the end of the nineteenth century much remained to be done, after decades which saw child labor reduced—but not eliminated. The efforts of Lord Shaftesbury, Mary Carpenter, and others saw advances in child welfare (Jordan 1998a–c), and the decades after 1870 saw education more firmly assured. However, at the end of the nineteenth century much remained to be done. The reformer and leader of the Salvation Army, William Booth, published in 1890, *In Darkest England and the Way Out*. In the pressing matter of families and their quality of life General Booth posed a challenge: "What then is the standard towards which we may venture to aim … it is the standard of the London Cab Horse … every Cab Horse in London has three things; a shelter for the night, food for its stomach, and work allotted to it by which it can earn its corn." Many children lacked Booth's three elements and were exposed to a number of threats to life and to survival. For sketches of London street children by John Leech in 1841 see Jordan (1992). Charles Dickens learned how hard life could be during his experience as a child worker in a factory, which made a product called Warren's Blacking. More oppressive to children's health and life was employment in heavy industry. This complex gave rise to the verbal label coined by William Blake—"the Dark Satanic Mills." The background was what Alexander Ure termed, The Mighty Moloch of Steam, referring to the visible power of steam engines as they energized the expanding factory system. Beyond the factory gates, the pace of social change had become differentiated into the growth of factory towns and the inversely deteriorating health of their populations (Jordan 1987a, b, 1993a, b).

Observing the paradox some denied the realities. For example, Ure published his *Philosophy of Manufactures* (1835), and insisted that, "... all the hard work is done by the steam-engine which leaves for the attendant no labour at all." On the other hand, Michael Sadler, Mary Carpenter, Lord Shaftesbury, Thomas Barnardo, Charles Booth and William Booth (unrelated), and other reformers across the century promoted reforming legislation as the means to protect working adults and children, and to expand education. For family life, a major item was Edwin Chadwick's report on sanitary conditions published in 1845. The Great Chadwick, as he is remembered, exposed the appalling accumulation of sewage and related threats to health. He demonstrated highly cost-effective ways to bring sanitation and clean water to households which, combined with initiatives in housing for ordinary families, reduced child mortality. Table 4.1 lists some of the events across the dynamic century which affected the lives of children.

It will be noted that the second item in Table 4.1 is the severe outbreak of scarlet fever in 1839—then a far more lethal strain than today's version. This disease spread from child to child in school then spread among brothers and sisters of the carrier. The same mechanism transmitted the great killer of the age, tuberculosis known then as phthisis, or consumption. In the early years of Victoria's long reign (1837–1901) "... deaths by consumption in London are double those of any other disorder," reported Dr. George Gregory (1840). Two years before, in 1838, William Farr had lost his young wife to that disease.

Density of population was a factor in this disease, and the century saw an increase in propinquity as the population per square mile rose across the decades; in 1831, there were 238 persons per square mile, a figure which rose to 558 persons per square mile in the 1901 Census.

In 1866, Farr, now the authority on public health statistics, identified premature birth at 4.49% as the principal cause of infant mortality; more surprising was the second cause, convulsion, at 3.50%. The term is vague, but appears to include symptoms traceable to premature weaning from the breast.

For little children diphtheria was always a risk to life, measles encephalitis was a possibility, and whooping cough was dangerous. It peaked in the epidemic of 1832–1834 in July and August (Farr 1866). The mechanism probably was a drop in the water table permitting pollution of sanitary devices. For infants, this was the

Table 4.1 The Victorian era: events influencing child welfare and mortality

Year	Event
1837	Registration of births and deaths in England and Wales
1839	Acute epidemic of scarlet fever in London
1840	Chimney sweeps act
1842	First report of the commission on the employment of children. Mean London January temperature −0.4°C
1844	Health of towns report
1845	Engel's *Condition of the working class in England*
1850s	Females 25–34 years: 49% of deaths due to tuberculosis
1851	Mayhew's *London labor and the London poor*
1854	Youthful offenders act. Dickens' *Hard Times*
1855	Committee on the adulteration of food established
1862	Lowe introduces "payment for results" into schools. little's monograph on cerebral palsy
1864	Registration of births and deaths in Ireland
1866	Fourth and final cholera epidemic in England
1867	4 lb. Wheat loaf costs 10.25 pennies
1868	Torrens' housing act
1869	Charity organzation society formed
1870	Forster's education act. Cross's artisans housing act. Barnardo's first home for children
1871	Illiteracy: males = 19.4%, females = 26.8%
1873	Bridges and Holmes issue, *proposed changes in hours and ages of employment …*
1878–1897	Very cold winters
1890	Salvation army's general booth issues, *in darkest england and the way out.* Child emigrants exceed 100,000
1890s	Measles mortality peaks
1891	Textile industry: workers under 15 years = 13.5%
1903	*Report of the interdepartmental committee on physical degeneration*

period of "summer fever" when infant mortality tended to rise. Another aspect of cleanliness was spread of typhus through insect bites when people did not wash; early twenty-first century travelers' worries about a resurgence of bedbugs seems reminiscent of earlier days. Smallpox was a threat, and to many it was a predictable and hazardous rite of childhood to be anticipated. Those not killed were likely to carry pox scars thereafter.

In his book of historic significance, *The Condition of the Working Class in England*, Friedrich Engels recorded that, "… in Manchester … more than 57% of the children of the working class perish before the fifth year, while but 20% of the children of the higher classes … die under 5 years." In 1866, Farr generalized the risk of death for the young in the age segment 0–5. He chose "30 large town districts," and "63 healthy districts." The average percentage of deaths in the thirty districts was 10.99%, but it was only 4.04% in the 63 districts he had previously chosen as healthy. The data from which these observations flow are themselves a matter of interest. The Benthamite utilitarians and census commissioners chose to report mortality using ages rather than dates of birth.

Mitchell (1971 et seq.) reported mortality data in the format 0–1, 0–4, 5–9 years, etc.; the earliest stages of life are important because they are the context of high rates of mortality. However, the 1837 initiative into recording births and deaths excluded stillbirths; in that regard, there is an unavoidable arbitrariness to defining age segments for the purpose of making records and specifications evolve; in 1992, "... the legal definition of a stillbirth was changed from a baby born dead after 28 or more weeks completed gestation to one born dead after 24 weeks ..." (Infant ... 2007).

With regard to the age segments of 5 years reported by Mitchell, that quinary permits consolidation of data and economies when developing graphs and schematic presentations. Alternatives might draw on biologically significant phases, such as adolescence; in such instances there would be gender differences to take into account. At the extreme of the age range, there are newer classifications such as "old old" for people over 85 years. In this book attention now turns to relating quality of life as formulated in the VICQUAL index to the rates of mortality for young children.

There is little information on the mortality associated with the end of gestation in the Victorian era. To place that era in perspective, consider that mortality rates at ages 0–4 in 1850 were 67 deaths per thousand live births (K) and there were 17 per thousand live births in 1938 (Mitchell 1971). The decline in mortality for little children was by a factor of five. The stillbirth rate in 2006 was five per one thousand births in England and Wales. The highest local rate of stillbirths in 2006 was 7.2 deaths per thousand, and it occurred in Anglesey, North Wales. Deaths in the first 4 years of life clearly are not stillbirths, but are used here as a numerical guide. It seems reasonable to speculate that stillbirths in the Victorian era occurred at an appalling rate, perhaps five times or more than of the mid-twentieth century.

4.3 Quality of Life

Changes in quality of life across the dynamic century and their implications for mortality among children evolved year by year throughout the Victorian era. The VICQUAL index numbers provide an estimate of the quality of life between Waterloo and the outbreak of the Great War, the era known as the Long Peace. This index draws on annual data from 14 variables in three domains. They are, economics, social matters, and health (Jordan 1993a, b); see Table 4.2.

Table 4.3 summarizes quinary data for mortality at three ages, male and female, and VICQUAL index numbers. The years 1847–1857 have the lowest index numbers, and illustrate persisting effects of the Hungry Forties. In the age group 0–9 years mortality index numbers for boys exceed those for girls. Also, mortality index numbers are higher among boys in 5–9 age group.

Table 4.2 Description of the VICQUAL source variables

Variable	Source
(Economic)	
Alcohol produces (Gal per capita)	Mitchell (1962)
Wage index	Mitchell (1975)
Commodity price index	Kondratieff (1926)
4 lb.-Loaf price (d.)	Mitchell (1962)
VICY Economic sub-index	Jordan (1992)
(Social)	
Birth Rate (per K)	Hunt (1981)
	Innes (1938)
	Griffith (1967)
Alcohol consumption per capita (gal.)	Wilson (1940)
Male literacy %	Vincent (1989)
Housing construction (K)	1911 Census (1917)
Rainfall (mm.)	Mitchell (1975)
(Health)	
Death rate (per K)	Mitchell (1958)
January F°	Drummond (1942)
Death Rate—TB (%)	Cronjé (1984)
Tea consumed (lb. per capita)	Mitchell (1962)

In 1838–1843, mortality rates for children of unspecified gender under one year averaged 150 deaths per one thousand live births; for the 5 years 1898–1902, the mortality rate for the group under one year was 152 deaths. The rate dropped briefly to 130 in 1881, having peaked in 1846 and 1847 at 164 deaths per one thousand live births.

The five highest mortality rates among males occurred between 1847 and 1870 and averaged 76.82 deaths per thousand. For girls, the five peak years fell between 1840 and 1866, and averaged 66.36 deaths per thousand. In the 5–9 age segment, the highest mortality rates were much lower. Among boys the five peak years fell between 1840 and 1863 and averaged 10.64 deaths per thousand. At 10.30 deaths per thousand, girls had a slightly lower rate.

For boys ages birth to four the peak rate of mortality was 77.80 in 1863, and among girls the peak rate of 67.50 deaths occurred twice, in 1854 and 1863. In the case of the 5–9 group, mortality was less frequent; among boys the peak rate 11.20 in 1849, and the girls the peak rate was 10.90 deaths in the same year, 1849.

The relationship between the VICQUAL index and children's mortality rates is amenable to various modes of presentation and analysis. Procedurally, both variables are reported in quinaries (i.e., sets of five); e.g., 1898–1902. VICQUAL index numbers use 1914 as the criterion, and mortality rates are indexed to 1902.

Pearson *r* correlations between annual VICQUAL index numbers and annual mortality rates are not statistically significant for children under one year ($r = 0.23$, *n.s.*). This indicates that the deaths of the youngest children across the period of interest appear to be, broadly speaking, statistically independent of the flow of events associated with the quality of life across the Victorian era Table 4.4.

Table 4.3 Child mortality in England and Wales: 1838–1902

Years	Quinary mortality index numbers (1902 = 100)					VICQUAL
	All	Males		Females		Index numbers
	<1 year	0–4	5–9	0–4	5–9	(1914 = 100)
1837–1842	102	115	126	84	46	99.18
1843–1847	100	116	207	95	50	95.83
1848–1857	96	117	226	83	46	95.79
1853–1857	100	117	195	83	52	102.11
1858–1862	101	116	205	83	53	97.96
1863–1862	99	121	202	80	54	101.62
1868–1872	99	116	191	85	56	105.15
1873–1877	104	110	155	89	69	110.99
1878–1882	108	105	149	94	71	107.18
1883–1887	107	101	128	98	79	101.15
1888–1892	106	100	103	100	89	101.60
1893–1897	101	100	103	99	96	101.80
1898–1802	101	100	95	103	102	107.08

Table 4.4 Correlations (*r*) between annual VICQUAL numbers and annual mortality rates of children, 1838–1902

Mortality rates				
<1 Year	0–4 Years		5–9 Years	
Male + Female	Male	Female	Male	Female
0.23	−0.28	−0.28	−0.45	−0.50
n.s.	0.05	0.05	0.001	0.0001

Significant correlations with the same numerical values obtained for both boys and girls in the age group 0–4 years ($r = 0.28$, $p = 0.05$). For this age, segment of both boys and girls expanded to age four, the years of highest mortality rates are narrow.

In the case of the oldest group of children, those ages 5–9 years, the correlation between VICQUAL index numbers and mortality data reached statistically significance: $r = -0.56$, and -0.58 ($p = 0.05$). The statistically significant negative values mean that the relationship between quality of life and mortality rates was inverse; as quality of life rose, mortality rates for children ages 5–9 declined. In view of the limited number of observations statistical significance does not automatically connote empirical significance, but it suggests a trend. However, for the age span of 0–9 years, in three segments, for boys and girls mortality becomes more influenced by the VICQUAL index of Victorian quality of life as the years of development pass.

When VICQUAL's variables in three domains (see Table 4.2) are combined the years from 1853 to 1857 are qualitatively superior. They occurred just before scarlet fever reached the first of four peaks of incidence, as Fig. 4.1 demonstrates.

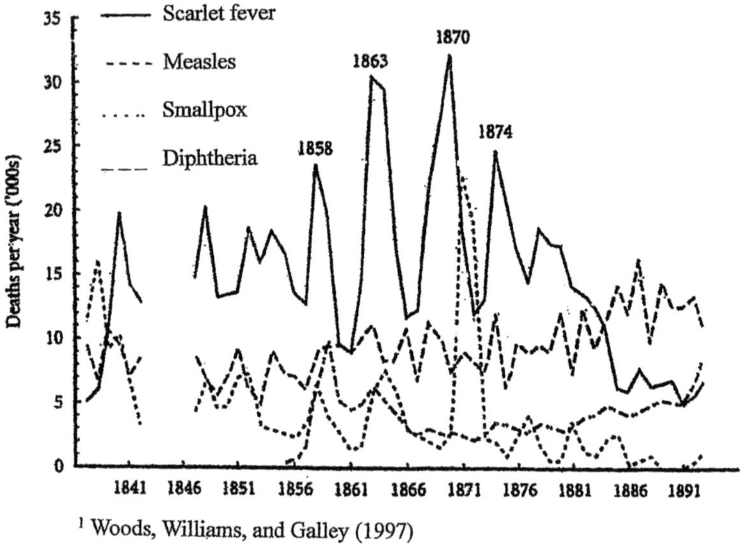

Fig. 4.1 Annual deaths from scarlet fever, measles, smallpox, and diphtheria, 1837–1892 (Woods et al. (1997))

The 10 years from 1868 to 1877 seem to have been comparatively favorable for children and adults, but scarlet fever reached its nineteenth century maximum in 1870, as did measles.

From Figure 4.1 it is evident that four communicable diseases were responsible for many deaths. Diphtheria slowly ended toward the last decade, and smallpox largely ended, as compulsory vaccination demonstrated its value. This last disease had seemed to earlier generations an inevitable risk of death to children; for them survival had its price; those who lived after infection sometimes bore sequelae in the form of facial scars and sensory problems Table 4.5.

This chapter draws on records of deaths across England Wales, a step not possible on a broad scale before the Victorian era and its Benthamite enthusiasms. Attention to improvement of civil records—at that point local parish registers which were incomplete and were prone to exclude nonAnglicans—began in 1777 with the innovations of the Rev. Mr. William Dade of St. Olave's parish in the diocese of York (Levene 2006). Finally, in 1874, civil registration in England and Wales became comprehensive with the registration of deaths, a step hailed by Woods (2000) as, "the shining star of Victorian civil registration."

Table 4.3 extracts from Mitchell (1971) years in which death rates for children were high and low. For three ages and both genders the years in which deaths per thousand live-born children were high spread across the decades addressed here; for babies, the mortality rate in 1899 was practically the same as in 1846, a high rate of 163 and 164 per thousand live births. For boys and girls at two ages, 0–4, and 5–9, the rates are much lower, and they are spread more narrowly.

Table 4.5 Age-specific death rates, high and low incidence per K England and wales 1838–1902

One year[a]		Males 0–4		5–9		Females 0–4		5–9	
Year	Rate	Year	Rate	Year	Rate	Year	Rate	Year	Rate
High incidence									
1846	164	1847	79.0	1840	10.8	1840	64.5	1840	10.6
1850	162	1849	75.0	1848	10.4	1846	66.7	1848	9.8
1865	160	1854	77.3	1849	11.2	1854	67.5	1849	10.9
1895	161	1863	77.8	1858	10.5	1863	67.5	1858	10.4
1899	163	1870	75.0	1863	10.3	1866	65.6	1863	9.9
Low incidence									
1845	142	1881	56.6	1886	4.8	1881	48.0	1898	3.9
1877	136	1883	61.0	1898	4.1	1883	51.1	1899	4.2
1879	135	1887	62.5	1897	3.9	1888	48.0	1900	4.2
1888	136	1894	56.1	1899	4.1	1894	47.4	1901	4.1
1902	133	1902	54.1	1902	3.9	1902	45.0	1902	4.2

Mitchell 1971
[a] Gender not specified

The years of comparatively low child mortality are also spread across the century. For the youngest children the best (lowest) rate is 142 per 1,000 in 1845, and by 1902 it had only declined a little. Four of the 5 years of low rates are in the final quarter-century. For boys in the age group 0–4, the last two decades show annual rates a little below the highest rates, and they begin in 1881. For boys 5–9 years, the lowest rates are about one-half of the highest rates, and they occurred in the same final two decades.

In the case of girls, the lowest rates are substantially below the highest rates, and a little below those for boys. For girls in the range 0–4 years, their best rates (i.e., low incidence) were fairly consistent across the last two decades, but not falling below 45 per 1,000 live births, but falling well below the worst rates of death. For the 5–9 group, the best rates, in the last 5 years, were well below the worst rates, and about one-half the rate.

The general impression is that child mortality fell across the course of the century, but with alarming exceptions as in the case of the infants and toddlers under one year at the time of their deaths. The annual rates for the group below one year were very high in the earliest years, and remained so across the nineteenth century. For boys and girls living long enough to be in the 5–9 age band, the rates declined substantially, and were still lower (but high by today's standards) and falling substantially.

The reality of life in nineteenth century Britain was caught in the aphorism that where wealth accumulates, there men decay. Oliver Goldsmith's Sweet Auburn evolved into the Dark Satanic Mills of William Blake, and until, decade by decade, working conditions—especially for children—became less inhumane.

In the files of the Registrar General, an office eventually occupied by Dr. William Farr, a man of humble origins (1807–1883), are city and county

Table 4.6 County mortality rates by age and gender, 1841

	Male		Female	
Rate	County	Incidence per K	County	Incidence per K
Ages 5–15 years				
Highest	Rutland	1.16	Rutland	1.12
Typical	Shropshire	0.74	Oxford	0.77
Lowest	Dorset	0.40	Westmorland	0.36

Calculated from Humphries 1991

mortality rates by age and gender (Humphries 1981); here, the gender mortality rates for ages 5–10 in 36 English counties are employed. For 1841, in the earliest years of Queen Victoria's long reign, the counties with the highest and lowest *female* mortality rates were tiny Rutland—1.12, and Westmoreland—0.36 per K. See Table 4.6. In the case of *males*, Rutland also had the highest rate of mortality, at 1.16 per K; the lowest county rate for males was in Dorset, at 0.40 per K. Typical counties, i.e., in the middle of the range, were (Males) Shropshire, and (Females) Oxfordshire.

Table 4.7 draws on Humphries' (1991) data to describe mortality rates in towns at two age segments, 5–10 years, and 10–15 years. For the 5–10 year group of females, Bristol was the most dangerous place, with a mortality rate in 1841 of 1.16 per K. Halifax posed the least threat among 38 towns with a mortality rate of 0.66; the lowest rate. For males, Liverpool was a dangerous place having a mortality rate of 1.74 per K, while the rate of mortality in Halifax was 0.65 per K. Towns with typical mortality rates were (Males) Derby, and (Females) Walsall. Among the young persons 10–15 years of age the rate of urban mortality was generally lower than that of the 5–10 group. For *females* the highest rate of urban mortality was in Macclesfield at 1.05 per K, and the lowest *male* rate among 50 towns was Yarmouth at 0.31 per K. For *males* Macclesfield had a high mortality rate of 1.05, which is virtually the same as that for *females*, see Table 4.7. The lowest *male* urban mortality rate was in Worcester—0.35 per K. Typical towns were (*male*) Colchester, and (*females*) Wakefield.

The death of the children was a frequent tragedy in the Victorian era. Infectious diseases claimed many lives, and among them were smallpox, measles, scarlet fever, and diphtheria—the latter pair being clearly distinguished in the last half of the century. Table 4.8 lists causes of death in boys and girls in three age groups. Scarlet fever was more fatal in boys, but in boys and girls it was more frequent in the 5–14 years group. Among children under one year "development and wasting" were the most frequently designated cause. Whooping cough was least likely in boys and girls 5–14 years. Influenza was an unlikely cause of death in boys and girls at all ages.

By age five bronchitis was unlikely to be a fatal illness, although the "respiratory system" was vulnerable up to age 4 years. For youngest children diarrhea and related conditions were highly dangerous; speculation has called attention to the choice not to breast-feed, and to the rise of prepared nutrients given by bottle.

Table 4.7 Urban mortality rates in two age groups by gender

Rate	Male		Female	
	County	Incidence per K	County	Incidence per K
Ages 5–10 years				
Highest	Liverpool	1.74	Bristol	1.16
Typical	Derby	1.12	Walsall	0.95
Lowest	Halifax	0.65	Halifax	0.66
Ages 10–15 years				
Highest	Macclesfield	1.05	Macclesfield	1.03
Typical	Colchester	0.73	Wakefield	0.66
Lowest	Worcester	0.35	Yarmouth	0.31

Calculated from Humphries 1991

Table 4.8 Diseases per 1,000 death in two age groups, by gender, 1848–1872

Disease	Males			Females		
	<1 Year	1–4 Years	5–14 years	<1 Year	1–4 Years	5–14 Years
Typhus	5	37	117	5	41	140
Smallpox	10	22	33	11	22	31
Measles	14	80	21	15	82	24
Scarlet fever	20	204	243	20	199	257
Whooping cough	34	63	11	46	88	17
Diphtheria	–	–	–	–	–	–
Influenza	2	2	1	2	2	2
Cholera	3	9	19	3	8	18
Dysentery	3	4	2	3	3	2
Tuberculosis, all forms	63	118	164	62	105	192
Convulsions	198	56	–	184	56	–
Nerv. system and senses	210	85	72	196	81	68
Cerebr. hem. apoplexy	3	5	9	3	4	8
Respiratory system	150	172	59	141	171	62
Bronchitis	59	60	15	57	61	16
Pneumonia	81	98	31	75	97	93
Digestive disorders	116	63	42	117	64	42
Dev'pm. and wasting	266	–	–	269	–	–
Prematurity	112	–	–	110	–	–

Source Logan 1950. Tables 3B & D., 3D, and #., 4B. and D

Cow's milk in an era before pasteurization raised the risk of spreading bovine tuberculosis. Such elements may be related to the fatal consequences of maternal illiteracy and lack of preparation for mothering. This complex was the agenda for reformers and for middle class mothers' efforts to prepare young women in the lower classes for motherhood and raising a family; fresh air and hygiene, for example, were among the themes promoted. It may be noted in passing that one of the arguments advanced by people opposed to the expansion of elementary schooling was the risk of spreading diseases by placing numbers of children in classrooms.

4.4 Discussion

The VICQUAL index estimates annual quality of life formulated from fourteen variables across the years of the Long Peace, an era which witnessed the rise of an imperial nation with a vibrant economy. Hegemony around the globe was recorded on maps in red, but it also was evident in the pale and wan complexions of Britons living within a nidus of factories and slums. The human cost of economic growth was evident in high mortality rates among the young.

Edwin Chadwick spoke of "generally assumed laws of a heavy mortality … applicable to every stage of infant life" (Chadwick 1844a, b). However, such generalizations have given way to increasingly particular models in which the objective is to identify the, "… many important factors that are difficult to measure with observed variables (which) may still constitute an important source of variation between individuals" (Bengtsson and Dribe 2010).

Correlating VICQUAL index numbers with child mortality rates assess the connection between quality of life and the persistent deaths of children. The range of $\underline{r}$'s in the five statistical relations ranged from 0.23 to −0.50 with the association for boys and girls in the age group 5–9 years reaching the 0.001 level of statistical significance. It seems realistic to consider the set of $\underline{r}$'s as a continuum. In that perspective children's mortality rates increasingly reflected the quality of life in England and Wales which rose in some respects while remaining deplorable in others, e.g., infant mortality. Child mortality was within a still wider concern to the Victorians. Around them they saw the consequences of urbanization and industrialization in the form of deteriorating health and habitus, and the prevalence of social ills (Jordan 1993b).

Attention shifts to the question of why the earliest years, those below age four, are less influenced by the increasing if selective improvements in quality of life, as measured by the VICQUAL index numbers. The 5–9 year-olds may be construed as survivors of a culling of their birth cohort evident in high rates of mortality at younger ages. The prospects for survival increased within a given birth cohort as children reached successive birthdays; they also increased as cohort succeeded cohort across the century, although the decline in mortality rates remained comparatively modest.

It is to cultural practices that we turn to elucidate the persistence of high mortality rates. Surmise suggests that there were elements in the Victorian way of life which were inimical to childhood, apart from the ever-present reach of a malign, or at best indifferent, Nature. Victors of death may be grouped as follows:

Society. Across the years of interest and well beyond the major risk to life for children had its origins in the inequities of social class; the poorest were at greatest risk, and those who reached adulthood had a shorter life expectancy. On the other hand, children of the privileged were no less susceptible to major diseases in an era before antibiotics.

In 1844, the Rev. James Clay reported from Preston that, "while the gentry lose only 17 1/2% of infant life, the operatives lose 55 1/2%." Clay concluded that, "If the infant population of the working class could have been reared amidst the advantages of food, air attention & c., … during the last 6 years, 3,034 children would have reached 5 years of age, who, as it is, have been swept away prematurely by disease."

In 1866, London endured its last outbreak of cholera. The mortality rate per thousand residents was 97 in the poverty-stricken parish of St. George-in-the East, but only 2 per thousand in fashionable Hanover Square in the west (Luckin 1977).

A major trend of the era was urbanization and the rise of factories. At the end of the nineteenth century the Manchester district, Angel Meadow, was a crowded slum. The poet Alfred Tennyson asked,

> Is it well that while we range with science glorifying in the time, City children soak and blacken, soul and sense, in city slime?

Angel Meadow housed seven thousand souls on 23 acres which is 212 persons per acre. The mortality rate for all ages in the 3 years 1898–1890 was three times the national average of 50.90 deaths per one thousand persons; young children probably were over-represented in the district's high mortality rate. In 1897, the Rev. J. E. Mercer noted, "We have to think of the children of the slums … Home life they have none. Not long ago I found the mother of a family lying dead, the younger children playing around the bed and turning up the sheets in curiosity to examine the body, and the elder girl washing up on a table near the bed, and leaning the pots against the mother's leg to drain … neglected from their birth, thrown on their own devices while still infants … insufficiently warmed, clothed, fed, what chance have they?"

In the Yorkshire town to the east, Leeds, builders emphasized the cheap back-to-back design in which fresh air was impeded; tuberculosis ran through those dwellings, as it had done in the nearby town of Haworth where it infected the family of the Rev. Mr. Patrick Bronte. Tuberculosis killed the poet John Keats and his brothers George and Thomas.

Table 4.9 demonstrates changes in the diets of families of rural laborers over the last four decades of the nineteenth century. (In Table 4.9 the "standard unit" is one farm laborer.) Use of sugar rose considerably, as did meat, and bread declined. Inclusion by Fussell (1929) of skimmed milk in the 1902 dietary, recorded an ill-advised innovation, the availability of skimmed milk. It was cheap and so appealing to the poor; however, in terms of nutrition it was, to use an old expression, "nowt but watter bewitched."

Across the nineteenth century there appeared a series of publications intended to offer guidance on family life and on ways to promote the health of children. In 1825 Esther Copley wrote *Cottage Comforts*, followed in 1849 by her *Cottage Cookery*. In 1879 there appeared *The Mother's Handbook: A Book for Her Own and Her Children's Management with Hints and Helps for Everyday Emergencies*. Of course, such documentary approaches presumed literacy and a middle class outlook unlikely to be present in the target audience. Even after Forster's (1870) law, the curriculum was slow to incorporate the real needs of children destined to become parents and to recycle familiar practices.

Table 4.9 Farm labourers' weekly dietaries

Item (in lbs.)	1863 Family	1863 Standard unit	1902 Family	1902 Standard unit
Bacon	4.55	1.2		
Total meat	4.55	1.2	7.15	1.9
Bread	55.75	14.7	38.83	10.2
Oatmeal and rice			1.25	0.3
Potatoes	27.0	7.1	25.75	6.8
Cheese	1.5	0.4	1.2	0.3
Butter, lard, margarine, and drippings	1.56	0.4	2.07	0.5
Tea, coffee, or cocoa	0.14		0.61	
Sugar (in pts.)	2.0	0.5	4.31	1.1
Milk: new skimmed	1.75	0.5	4.5 or 8.75	1.2 or 2.3

Source Adapted from Fussell (1929)

One of the philanthropic movements of the nineteenth century was the Ladies Sanitary Association whose home visitors advised young mothers on how to raise their children. The lady visitors advocated fresh air, cleanliness, and good nutrition. The Association issued tracts.

THE SICK CHILD'S CRY
Open the window, Mother,
I can't breathe in this stifling room;
Open the window, Mother,
And let out the weight and gloom !
(Jordan 1987a, b)

Balance requires acknowledgment of the place of reformers such as the Grant brothers in Lancashire, memorialized by Dickens as the Cheerybles. In Yorkshire, near Halifax, the industrialist Edward Akroyd began to build Akroydon's model housing; near Leeds Titus Salt built Saltaire. Such housing initiatives were a shrewd blend of amelioration of quality of life, control of the labor force, and cupidity, along the lines of the housing built in Germany by Alfred Krupp.

4.4.1 Family

The dynamics of family life and the quality of parenting skills influenced the survival of children, then as now. Among the working poor there was the practice of ensuring that the breadwinner was well fed, and mother and children came second. Food itself was a hazard to health. Bakers adulterated their product in several ways. Alum was used to blanch brown grains (Odling 1857). Families which provided milk for their children paradoxically placed them at risk. Milk was adulterated with water of uncertain purity; milk also presented the risk of transmitting bovine tuberculosis.

According to Smith (1988), post-mortem examinations in the 1880s on 1,420 children, nominally dying from a variety of illnesses, revealed an incidence of tuberculosis in 30% of them.

Within families seeking respite from a crying baby there was recourse to a variety of sedatives. Mother's Friend, Poppy Tea, Dalbey's Carminative, and Godfrey's Cordial (Jordan 1987a, b) were based on the juice of the poppy we know as heroin. Caretakers feeding Mrs. Wilkinson's Soothing Syrup to infants placed them in a sleep from which they might not awaken. Those who survived persistent sedation appeared pale, "feeble and usually die, seldom completing the second year," reported Friedrich Engels (1845).

Illegitimate and otherwise "inconvenient" infants placed in the care of baby-farmers, slipped into a deep and endless sleep. In his essay on baby-farming the Rev. Mr. Bejamin Waugh recorded that for 50 pounds a woman guaranteed that an inconvenient fetus would not be born alive. Baby-farming was a shadowy and sinister trade.

The rise across the decades in the level of material life was slow, and it was not uniformly beneficial. Life expectancy increased, but only among those who survived the destruction of young lives. For the most vulnerable, amelioration of cultural threats to life evolved through legal steps, and through personal reforms within family life.

References

Bengtsson, T., & Dribe, M. (2010). Quantifying the family frailty effect in infant and child mortality by using median hazard ratio (MHR). The case of rural Sweden, 1766–1895. *Historical Methods, 43*, 15–27.

Census of England and Wales, 1911. (1917). London: His Majesty's Stationery Office.

Chadwick, E. (1828). Diminution of sickness and mortality. *Westminster Review, 17*, 355–421.

Chadwick, E. (1844a). On the best modes of representing accurately, by statistical returns, the duration of life, and the pressure and progress of the causes of mortality amongst the populations of different districts and countries. *Quarterly Journal of the Statistical Society of London, 7*, 1–40.

Chadwick, E. (1844b). Report on the sanitary condition of the laboring population of Great Britain. *Parliamentary Papers, 3*, 1–457.

Crowther, M. R. (1981). *The workhouse System 1834–1929*. London: Methuen.

Drummond, H. J. (1942). Cold winters at kew observatory, 1783–1942. *Quarterly Journal of the Royal Meteorological Society, 69*, 17–32.

Engels, F. (1845). *The condition of the working class in England*. London: Penguin.

Farr, W. (1866). Mortality of children in the principal states of Europe. *Journal of the Statistical Society, 29*, 1–39.

Fussell, G. E. (1929). Changes in farm labourers' diet during two centuries. *Economic History, 1*, 268–274.

Gregory, G. (1840). Statistics of mortality and disease in London. *Lancet*. 79-90.

Griffith, G. T. (1967). *Population Problems in the age of malthus*. New York: Kelly.
Heywood, J. (1839). Report of an enquiry, conducted from house to house, into the state of 176 families in Miles Platting, within the borough of Manchester. *Transaction of the Royal Society of London, 1*, 34–36.
Humphries, J. (1991). "Bread and a pennyworth of treacle": Excess female mortality in England in the 1840s. *Cambridge Journal of Economics, 15*, 451–473.
Hunt, E. H. (1981). *British labour history 1815–1914*. London: Weidenfeld and Nicholson.
Infant and perinatal mortality 2006: Health areas, England and Wales. (2007). *35*.
Innes, J. W. (1938). *Class Fertility Trends in England and Wales 1876–1934*. Princeton, NJ. Princeton University Press.
Jordan, T. E. (1987a). *Victorian Childhood: Themes and Variations*. Albany, NY. State University of New York Press.
Jordan, T. E. (1987b). "The Keys of Paradise": Godfrey's cordial and children in Victorian Britain. *Journal of the Royal Society of Health, 107*, 19–22.
Jordan, T. E. (1992). Children of the mobility: A street-level view of early Victorian children. *Journal of the Royal Society of Health, 112*, 25–30.
Jordan, T. E. (1993a). "L'Homme Moyen": Estimating the quality of life for British adults 1815–1914, an index. *Social Indicators Research, 29*, 183–203.
Jordan, T. E. (1993b). *The Degeneracy Crisis and Victorian Youth*. Albany, NY. State University of New York Press.
Jordan, T. E. (1998a). *The census of Ireland, 1821–1911*. Lewiston: Mellen. Three volumes.
Jordan, T. E. (1998b). *Ireland's children: Quality of life, stress, and child development in the famine era*. Westport: Greenwood.
Jordan, T. E. (1998c). *Victorian child savers and their culture: A thematic evaluation*. Lewiston: Mellen.
Jordan, T. E. (2011a). Whitelaw's essay on the population of Dublin (1805): A window on eighteenth century housing. *New Hibernia Review, 15*, 9–18.
Jordan, T. E. (2011b). Whitelaw's essay on the population of Dublin (1805): A window on late eighteenth century housing. *New Hibernia Review, 25*, 136–145.
Kelly, M., & O Grada, C. (2011). The poor law of old England: Institutional innovation and demographic regimes. *Journal of Inter Disciplinary History, 41*, 339–366.
Kondratieff, N. (1926). Die langen wellen der konjunktur. *Archiv fur Sozialwissenschaft und Sozialpolitik, 56*, 573–609.
Lee, C. H. (1991). Regional inequalities in infant mortality in Britain, 1861–1971: Patterns and hypotheses. *Population Studies, 45*, 55–65.
Levene, A. (2006). What can dade registers tell us about infant mortality in later eighteenth century? *Local Population Studies, 76*, 31–42.
Logan, W. P. D. (1950). Mortality in England and wales from 1848–1947. *Population Studies, 4*, 132–178.
Luckin, W. (1977). The final catastrophe—Cholera in London, 1866. *Medical History, 21*, 32–43.
Mayhew, H. (1851). *London labour and the London poor*. In P. Quennell (Ed.), *Mayhew's London*. New York: Spring Books (1969).
Mitchell, B. R. (1958). *British historical statistics*. Cambridge: Cambridge University Press.
Mitchell, B. R. (1962). *Abstract of British historical statistics*. Cambridge: Cambridge University Press.
Mitchell, B. R. (1971). *Abstract of British historical statistics*. Cambridge: Cambridge University Press.
Mitchell, B. R. (1975). *European historical statistics 1750–1970*. New York: Macmillan.
Odling, W. (1857). On the composition of bread. *Lancet, 1*, 137–138.
Quennell, P. (1969). *Mayhew's London*. New York: Springer.
Reid, A. (1977). Locality or class ? spatial and social differentials in infant and child mortality in England vand Wales. In C. Corsini & F. Viazzo (Eds.), *The Decline of Infant and Child Mortality: The European Experience*. The Hague: Nijhoff.

Sadler, M. (1833). *The justice, humanity, and policy, of restricting the hours of children and young persons in the mills and factories of the United kingdom.* Inchbold: Leeds.
Smiles, S. (1880). *Duty: With illustrations of courage, patience, and endurance.* New York: Allison.
Smith, F. B. (1988). *The retreat of tuberculosis, 1850–1950.* London: Croom Helm.
Vincent, D. (1989). *Literacy and popular culture: England 1750–1914.* Cambridge: Cambridge University Press.
Wilson, G. B. (1940). *Alcohol and the nation.* London: Nicholson and Watson.
Woods, R. (2000). *The demography of Victorian England and wales.* Cambridge: Cambridge University Press.
Woods, R., Williams, N., & Galley, C. (1997). Differential mortality patterns among infants and other young children: The experience of England and Wales in the nineteenth century. In P. Corsinu & P. Viazzo (Eds.), *The decline of infant and child mortality. The European experience.* Geneva: UNICEF.

Chapter 5
Birth, Life, and Death in Dublin, 1619–1798

The Reformation reached Ireland, effectively, in 1541 when the Dublin parliament re-named Ireland as a kingdom, and Henry VIII became both king and head of the church. His designated Archbishop had influence within the Pale, and under the two Tudor sisters, Mary and Elizabeth, the new theology waned and waxed under aggressive religio-political enthusiasms. In the 1640s O'Neil's uprising and the subsequent repression under Oliver Cromwell led to consolidation of English Protestant hegemony and expulsion of Dublin's Catholics. Compounding, the population changes were outbreaks of plague as the victors consolidated their gains.

As a whole, seventeenth century Dublin was a walled city whose space grew a little across the century; the river Liffey and its soft banks at Ringsend ended where the tributary Dodder finished its northward flow. The Liffey was increasingly enclosed by quays which created land and provided space for buildings and roads. A bridge connected the south bank to the area which had been home to Norsemen, and which was served by St. Michan's parish; see Fig. 5.1. Dublin's population grew across the century from about 6,000 residents to over 70,000 (Butlin 1965). In time, St. Michan's was supplemented by two other parishes.

Evolution sometimes occurred in the form of consolidation; an example, in what is now north Dublin city, combined the parishes of St. Margaret, St. Canice, St. Nicholas, and St. Bridget, at Finglas (Ni Mhurchadha 2007). Similarly, St. Bridget's was combined with St. Stephen and St. Michael le Pole parishes. Another example of parish evolution is the separation of St. Catherine and St. James in 1707 (Gillespie 2004). Finally, there is evolution in the form of resurrection; there is the suppression, then the rebirth of the ancient parish of St. Andrew in 1666 (Gillespie 2004).

From their medieval roots Dublin's parishes in the seventeenth century provided housing crowded in narrow lanes for a polyglot population. From England came Protestant migrants and to a lesser degree came Scots Presbyterians who favored nearby Ulster. More exotic were Dutch entrepreneurs and French Huguenots and

T. E. Jordan, *Quality of Life and Mortality Among Children*,
SpringerBriefs in Well-Being and Quality of Life Research,
DOI: 10.1007/978-94-007-4390-8_5, © The Author(s) 2012

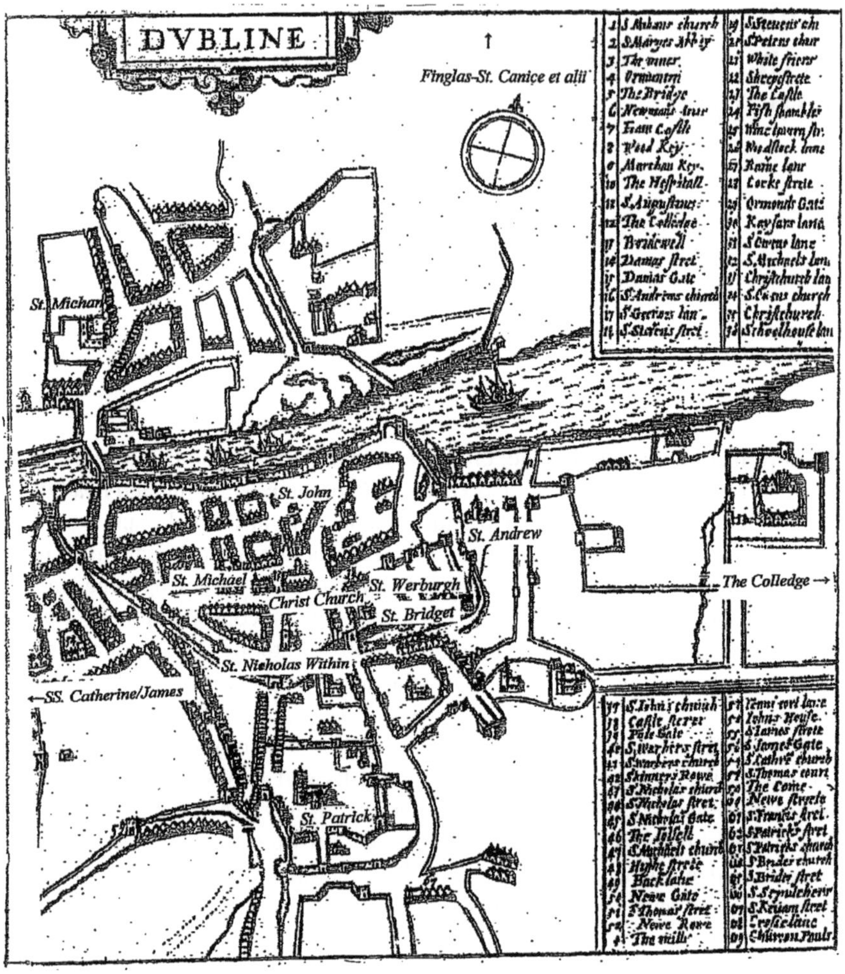

Fig. 5.1 Dublin parishes, seventeenth century

diaspora Jews. Forming other sectarian groups within the Protestant majority were Quakers fleeing persecution in England, and Baptists. Flight also shaped the demography of the city and its hinterlands. At mid-century, Protestants fled Dublin in the early 1640s and, in the next decade, Catholics were expelled from the city. They formed refugee encampments, and to the east of Dublin there appeared Irishtown, a name applied to settlements adjacent to other towns, e.g., Kilkenny.

Dublin's population is glimpsed in its parishes which fluctuated as their populations reflected intracity migrations. At one point, St. Michan's north of the Liffey became fashionable, and its quality of life rose. Similarly, the city government laid out St. Stephen's Green around which those of the privileged who did not settle in the suburbs built fine houses. Much of the city's wealth came from trade built on importing and exporting commodities such as fish, timber, and animal products. Dublin acted as an entrepôt for goods bought and sold beyond the Pale (Butlin 1977). Its harbor had sandbanks leading Dr. Gerald Boate to observe that,

> This haven, besides its shallowness, hath yet another great incommodity, that the ships have hardly any shelter there forv any winds ... as with a great southwest storm the ships run great hazards to be carried away from their anchors ... which more than once came to pass ... in the beginning of November, An. 1637, when in one night ten or twelve barks had that misfortune befall them ... whereof never no news hath been heard since (Jordan 2006).

Dublin had two political centers; one was the Tholsel, built on the site of the graveyard at St. Nicholas Within (Mills 1911) and the site of municipal government; the other was the Castle, a structure which was improved under the Lord Lieutenant, the ill-fated Thomas Wentworth.

Closer to the lives of Dubliners was the parish; originally a religious institution providing devotions its functions evolved to include charities, and its rolls provided a useful is somewhat limited roster of the inhabitants, chiefly for taxation such as the *cess*. This chapter draws on parish registers to consider life and death in Dublin's parishes across the seventeenth century.

Survival of ancient parish registers was largely a matter of indifference to their future value. The Proctor's records at St. Werburgh's, "languished for centuries in no particular order in a parish chest in the vestry ..." (Empey 2009). Keeping records of financial transactions, marriages, baptisms, and burials had been authorized in 1617 in an Office of Public Register, a function called for later in the century by Sir William Petty on several occasions—and an office he sought to fill himself. The 1617 law called for a fee of sixpence for the authorized functions. Such record-keeping and payment of fees was, in the idiom of the era, farmed out to an entrepreneur to collect money and to report the finances annually (Mills 1906). Had the registers and records been assembled as a single corpus they probably would have been placed in the archives at the Four Courts which burned in 1922.

Much of the credit for the existence of the parish records goes to the Parish Register Society of Dublin's activities in the first decade of the twentieth century. From the parish registers which the Society conserved, and from later publications, it is possible to examine births and deaths at two levels. Table 5.1 provides a numerical account of people as groups in eleven parishes; (it will be followed by a more focused consideration of several extant registers and their entries on life and death). The era analyzed in Table 5.1 is the last half of the seventeenth century; it should be borne in mind that parish registers, while generally maintained conscientiously, are not like census documents in their level of detail.

The average number of families known to parish officials was 375.90; depending on the multiplier applied to that figure, the total number residents varies. On the basis of five residents in a family the average parish sheltered 1,650 persons. When a multiplier of seven is applied the average parish had 2,351

Table 5.1 Parish characteristics, 1670–1695

				% 1 or 2 hearths		"good" housing[a]
Parish	Families	Births	Burials[1]	1664	1695	1695
St. Andrew/Donabrook	483	108	178	48	21	78
St. Bridget	416	70	100	30	14	80
St. Michan	656	127	221	60	20	72
SS Catherine/James	661	161	190	72	29	79
St. Michael	140	44	59	40	4	87
St. Nicholas within	93	28	34	44	3	96
St. Nicholas without	490	207	262	80	30	84
St. John	244	70	138	30	14	81
St. Werburgh	267	54	108	40	9	85
St. Audoens	216	53	121	49	21	72
Christ church	29	0	1	–	12	76
Mean	335.90	83.82	128.36	49.30	16.09	80.91
Total	3,695	922	1,412			

Jordan 2010a, b, c

[a] "Tenanted by people of some condition" (Butlin 1965)

residents. Christ Church was the exception since it was home to the celibate professors at Trinity College (see Fig. 5.1). In terms of population, the largest and smallest parishes were St. Michan and St. Nicholas Within—excepting Christ Church.

More central is the population dynamic of births and deaths in Dublin, acknowledging that not every such event was formally recognized. Butlin 1965 typified calculating the population as a "task fraught with difficulty." It is evident from Table 5.1 that there was serious imbalance between births and deaths, and that births—here approximated by baptisms—failed to replace the operant level of the population in all parishes. The mean values in Table 5.1 indicate that the replacement level was only 63.50%. As late as 1680, deaths exceeded births 1,826–1,096, and excess of 730 persons. To a degree mortality probably depended on the socio-economic level of families and their corresponding quality of life (Jordan 2010a, b, c); that is, the poorest were at greater risk to health and survival, although the state of peoples' health was not mitigated by effective medical care when plague and other diseases swept the city.

Table 5.1 lists the percentages of houses with only one or two hearths—an indicant of deprivation. The table indicates that in 1664 such impoverishment was most evident in the parish of St. Nicholas Without, and least in St. Bridget's. Three decades later, the number residences with two or one hearths had fallen considerably indicating a rising quality of life; St. Nicholas Without experienced the greatest change. In the same year, 1695, 80% of the parishes' housing was considered "good" by the standards of the times.

The second mode of inquiry into life and death derives from the registers directly. Parishes varied in the form their physical documents took. At St. Kevin's the register was a book of 476 paper sheets each 12 by 7 inches. However, a second volume consisted of 118 folios 15 inches square made from parchment and divided into three columns (Jordan 1993b). The register at St. Michan's conserved by Berry (Berry 1907) consisted of four volumes each of which was different. Volume 1 consisted of 37 sheets of parchment folios 15 by six and a half inches. Volume 2 was much larger and consisted of 889 pages. Volume 3 was 107 folios eleven and a half by 8 inches. Volume 4 had 340 folios of paper 16 by nine and half inches. In the case of SS. Catherine and James conserved by Gillespie 2004 the register was a "paper manuscript" of 381 pages in some disorder. An example of a parish register's page is given in Fig. 5.2, which is taken from the register at Finglas from 1661 to 1662.

The register at St. John the Evangelist consisted of two parchment documents the first of which was 12 by 11 inches. The second volume of 131 parchment sheets was twelve and one half by 12 and 3 quarter inches (Mills 1906). Empey 2009 found that the register at St. Werburgh's consisted of 83 folios.

The lives of parish residents had their origins, for the most part, in marriages celebrated in church. At the time, weddings were formal, and occurred after the banns had been read on "three Lord's Dayes"; they might be conducted by the resident minister, but there were occasions when parish officials presided. An example was the wedding of Richard Smith and Margarett Phillipps conducted at St. Michan's by "mee Captaine William Every one of the Justices of the Peace in the County of Dublin." Witnesses tended to be members of the parish vestry. One such witness was John Tadpole who also held a municipal office supervising the Searchers—"elderly matrons sworn to their duty," who recorded details of deaths for the Bills of Mortality.

Parish registers reflected the social status of the participants. In 1619 the Clarke at St. John the Evangelist, Bartholomew Jordane, recorded simply that Richard Browne and Mary Woott were married in February on an unspecified day, as were Nathaniell Hamon and Susan Prudfott a few days later. In contrast, the record was more complete in the case of "Sr Gustaves Humes Knight and Alice Morespinster dauaghter of the Right Honn^{ble} Henry More Earl of Droghedah, by the Reuerend John Pooley Dean of Kilkenny and prebendary of this parish of St. Michans pursuant to a Lycense issued out of the Prerogtive Court."

In the case of "H John Dauis Esqre and Ann Caulfild spinster daughter of the Ld Viscount Charlemount" the marriage ceremony was listed in the register at St. Michan's as performed by "the Right Reuend Nathaniel Foy Ld Bipp of Waterford," by the Prebendary, J. Clayton. (In these examples the original letter *u* is the equivalent of today's *v*.)

In the normal course of the marriage cycle births would follow in due season, and christenings were entered into parish registers. In the context of this consideration christenings are an indicant of births, rather than a measure or accurate number; the reasons are that not every birth was called to the attention of parish authorities, and those registered were members of the Established church. Catholics generally chose not to participate in the functions of the now firmly Protestant authorities. In that regard, however, Catholics served as sidesmen at Finglas at a time when such offices could be burdensome (Ni Mhurchadha 2007).

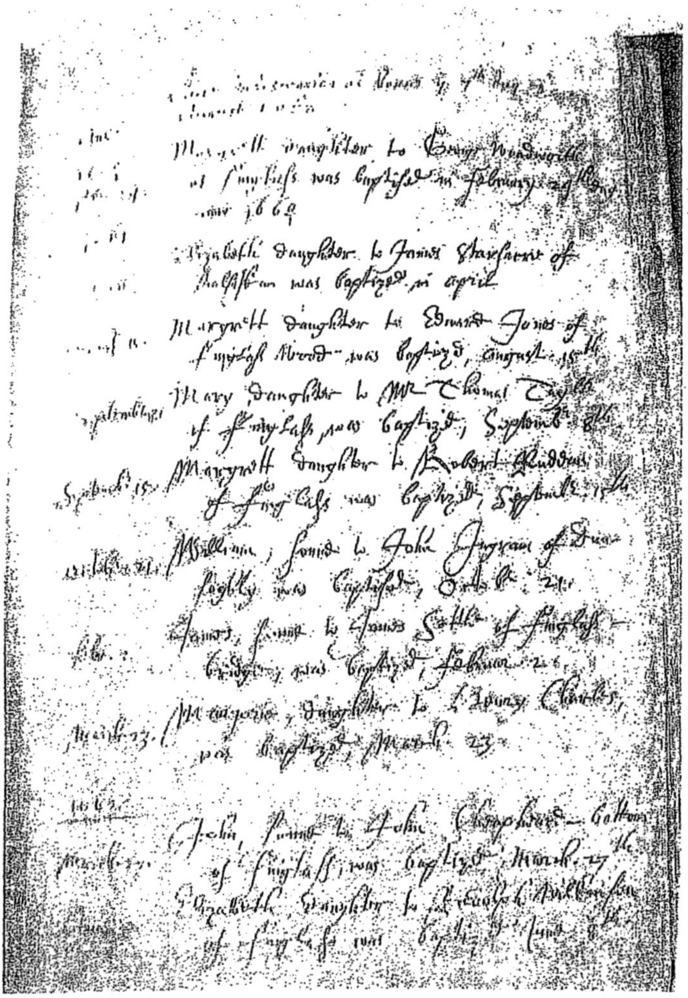
[1]Ni Mhurchadha, M. (2007). The Vestry Records of the United parishes of Finglas, St. Margaret's, Artane and the Ward, 1657 – 1758. Dublin. Four Courts Press.

By permission. ©Representative Church Body, Dublin.

Fig. 5.2 A page from the vestry records at Finglas. Ni Mhurchadha (2007). By permission. © Representative Church Body, Dublin

Dublin's parish registers provided information about one source of population replacement—native births among Dubliners. The other source of replacement was migration from the hinterlands, and the more extended hegira pursued by migrants from England.

Parish births were recorded in a fashion which shed light on the appalling death rate among the young. In Table 5.1 the births and burials show that births alone did not provide replacements. At St. Michan's 94 additional births were necessary in order to balance births and deaths. On the other hand, the small parish of St. Nicholas Within needed only six extra births in order to achieve replacement. Eventually, the in-migrants contributed to population balance and, to the population increases evident across the century.

Parish registers do not list age of the deceased. At St. John's on 11 December 1634, there was, "buried John ye sonne of Jams Tamson." In such instances John might have been a child or an adult. On the other hand, being a child could be explicit; in 1618–1619, St. John's register noted, "Y^{e} burial of Mr. Eaten's child" (Mills 1906). More detail was recorded for "Margarett Panckerman the daughter of Peter Panckerman was buryed the 23th day of April, 1660 (a child)," at St. Michan's. In the following year, a boy—possibly an adolescent—was interred: "John Reyly the sonne of John Reyly apprentice to Nicholas Wallis was buryed the 26th day of May, 1661."

Noticeable across the parishes are the burials of small children without names. In January 1641, St. John's recorded the interment of "a poor child," and in the following month another unnamed child's death; however, the register also noted a little more information on "Edward a poore child." We know a little more about these and other deaths; the register began its sad list with the heading, "The Names of ye poore English who having fled to this Citie for refuge and Dyed in ye parish of St. Johns …"

A double tragedy in 1622, at St. John's was, "… the burial of Besswoods daughters childe," and "the burial of Besswoods sonne." Perhaps the Besswoods lost both a son and a granddaughter in a single event, e.g., an epidemic.

At St. Catherine's, in 1685, the register was quite forthcoming in its record of the death of an infant, Ann. She was the tenth child of Thomas and Ann Bennett. This infant was baptized on "ye 11th of June, 1685, and buried ye 17th of August following," after 36 days of life.

Later that year, the parish interred "Mr Brown's child from New Row, 9," identifying one of the parents but not the child. More informative was the burial at St. Kevin's of "Thomas, sonn of Christopher Terry of New Rowe vpon the Pottle." In the following year St. Stephen's parish burial ground appears to have been used for the poor. The register recorded "A poore man and two poore girls bur. In St. Steph^{ns} Courtyard"; by that date, St. Stephens had been combined with St. Kevin and St. Peter parishes for 5 years. More unusual, some years later was the burial of "a Blackamore boy from Baron Worth's." At SS. Catherine and James the fee for a burial was 6 shillings and eightpence (£.33).

The death of poor children was more likely since they were at risk of abuse. In the case of one infant, the Vestry at SS. Catherine and James, in April 1660, insisted that the child assigned to Luke Lowther be presented to them alive in order to continue payments—"if shee live so long." One such child was Henry Street who was buried at SS. Peter and Kevin in November 1676; "Henry Street, one of the poore children wch had allowance from the pish." It is likely that the name,

Street, describes where the infant was found, which was the custom of the time. Similar is the name of an infant buried at St. Catherine's who appears to have been given the name of a street sign, "ye talbert in Thomas Street" (Parish 1908). It might seem that children once interred left mortal gaze forever; such is not the case. At St. Michan's whose crypt has soil with preservative properties, a child carefully dressed and buried in 1679 was found in the late nineteenth century. A preserved adult corpse may still be viewed in the crypt.

Dublin parishes continue to emerge as scholars bringing the contents of registers to light (Wallace 2011). Apart from the facts of life and death discussed in this chapter the registers are an archive of social data giving context to the bare facts. From St. Michan's come occupations unfamiliar today. A *Translator* converted wornout shoe leather into useable items. A *Gabbertman* steered the small boats carrying goods from Dublin Bay into the quays along the Liffey. A *Cleave* man carried baskets. A *Heyler* laid tiles, and a *Slaymaker* made parts for a loom (Berry 1907). Mills (1911) listed a *Ballore* as the parish crier. Empey 2009study of St. Werburgh's registers lists a *Dawber* as a plasterer, and a *Lavender* did laundry. A *Grote* was four pennies, and a *Furnyal* was a bakehouse.

Parishes added civil functions in time, and the register at St. Catherine's recorded, "A true returne of the number of all Hearthes firing places and stones publique ovens and kilns wthin the County of the Citty of Dublin for the yeare beginning the 25 day of March 1666 and … 25th day of March 1657." Patrick Ferell had four hearths and one oven on which the tax was 10 shillings (£.50). Mr. William Brookes (whose appellation, Mr. was an indicator of status) has "ffourteen hearths," and was assessed 28 shillings (£1.40). The register at Finglas (Ni Mhurchadha 2007) recorded a mode of providing for the poor. The privilege of begging within the parish required that the beggar wear a blue coat and display an official badge.

In later decades of the seventeenth century seating was introduced and generated sensitivities about rank. At St. Michan's there were fewer seats than worshipers, and a seat was shared by John Clotworthy—styled Lord Massereene sine 1660—and his social equal, Sir Michael Cole.

The register at SS. Peter and Kevin revealed human frailty; in 1670, a Churchwarden stole 12 pounds after having served only "aboute halfe a yeare," and fled to England. Registers also recorded quite mundane transactions as when the Vestry at Finglas, "paid to Jhon (sic) Rely for towards mending the Roofe of the Church," ten shillings and sixpence.

The seventeenth century registers of Dublin's parishes place the life cycle of people in all walks of life in perspective. The young died in great numbers, and the lives of all were in jeopardy when epidemics struck. Such events occurred against a background of rapid and violent social change. People sought recourse in the solace of religion amidst a variety of sectarian convictions. For all confessions, the centrality and familiarity of death created a theme of personal loss shared by all.

Life in eighteenth century Ireland saw population living out the implications of the preceding century and its tumultuous episodes. As that century ended the events of 1688, and the eclipse of hope among the people attendant to the Fall of the Catholic James II, set the stage for the next century. In particular, the restrictions on political life and civil rights suppressed possible moves to alleviate the condition of the people. What consideration of the quality of life occurred was overshadowed by erruptions of violence based on the appalling quality of life within the largely rural population.

As the eighteenth century opened Ireland had few centers of population, apart from regional sites such as Cork, Galway City, and Limerick. Dublin on the eastern shore continued to grow acting as an entrepôt for the island as a whole, and attracting migrants from the hinterlands. It did so at a time when the population exceeded the housing resources of the town, and only the rich could take advantage of uncongested areas in what today are suburbs. Dublin's choreography consisted of a series of parishes mostly south of the river Liffey. Parishes were no longer merely ecclesiastical units having taken up civic functions and working with the city's government. Relevant to consideration of mortality among children was the duty of parish vestries to bury children found dead on the streets, and to provide for the welfare of those still alive when discovered.

The final decade of the eighteenth century in Ireland was unsettled. James Napper Tandy had founded the Dublin branch of the United Irishmen in 1791, and tensions spread across the decade culminating in the events of 1798. In the years which followed the Act of Union in 1801 ended "Grattan's Parliament" in Dublin, and created the Westminster parliament as the locus of legislation for Ireland.

As the eighteenth century drew to an end the capacity of Dublin's parishes to cope with their social problems was overwhelmed. Housing, with its correlates of communicable disease, mortality, and family stress was insufficient, and amenities for disposal of human and material waste were rare. Noxious fumes were everywhere, and that at a time when vapors—*miasma*—were considered victors of disease.

These matters concerned the rector of the poor parish of St. Catherine in southwest Dublin. The Rev. James Whitelaw reflected on his impression of conditions in his parish which housed 20,000 people living on just over 100 acres; he decided to undertake a survey of all the housing in the city of Dublin. The city's old core of housing stock, he discovered, had changed little in over a century. Within the old city boundaries he counted 1,179 houses, a number exceeding Sir William Petty's count in 1682 by only 30 houses. In 1798 Whitelaw counted 16,023 houses in Dublin city. The work of Whitelaw and his assistants in the unusually hot summer of 1798 was facilitated to a degree by an impression among the poor—erroneous but helpful—that the door-to-door survey was preparatory to a scheme of relief.

Whitelaw produced a set of five hundred tables describing in great detail the condition of Dublin's housing and identifying by name, gender, and occupation—the inhabitants. This degree of detail is thought by some to have had a political aspect given the temper of the times, and the fact that the product in two volumes was immediately taken up by the Lord Lieutenant of Dublin Castle.

Whitelaw's two volumes with their lists of family circumstances are not available to us having perished in the civil was of 1922. Fortunately, Whitelaw composed a third element which he named an *Epitome*. From that source it is possible to draw inferences about mortality among children engulfed in an appalling quality of life. A house in a typical parish, say St. Andrew's or St. Mark's, had four floors and housed up to 15 people of all ages. Rooms were rented singly to families. Whitelaw observed:

> A single apartment in one of these truly wretched habitations, rates from one to two shillings per week; and to lighten the rent, two, three, and even four families, become joint tenants. I have frequently surprised from ten to sixteen persons, of all ages and sexes, in a room not fifteen feet square, stretched on a wad of filthy straw, swarming with vermin, and without any covering, save the wretched rags that constitute their wearing apparel.

Whitelaw encountered a house in School House Lane whose front wall has entirely fallen away leaving rooms exposed to the elements, but the rent collector showed up on Saturday night to collect the usual rent.

Table 5.2 reproduces Table XIV from Whitelaw's *Epitome*; the numbers yield a mean density per house of 9.67 persons; familiar names in the table are Dawson Street, Merion row, and Grafton street, among others.

The central topic of mortality is illuminated by O Grada (1991). From his analysis of mortality among babies born at the Rotunda hospital in the decades shortly after Whitelaw's work, O Grada placed mortality among children under 6 years at one-half, which is a typical rate for England and Ireland until the end of the nineteenth century.

Table 5.2 presents an *epitome*, to employ Whitelaw's term, of one parish which lists streets, people by gender (but not age), and the number of houses—with a note on their condition. The term "waste" was not defined by Whitelaw but, given the account of the fallen-down house in School House Street which remained occupied and rented, it probably was applied to houses below even that level of occupancy.

St. Anne's was an area of 63 standard acres and 7,228 souls in what is now central Dublin adjacent to St. Stephen's Green. Table 5.2 lists 35 streets and alleys containing 747 houses of which 36 were, in Whitelaw's term, "waste." The balance between the genders was markedly tilted toward females by about one-third. Streets and alleys varied in density, broadly speaking; that is, we know what 12 people live on the west side of Lower Merion Street, while Dawson Street sheltered 269 people; not available is the length of streets which would permit a more detailed appraisal.

It is possible to extract an impression of life in the city at an overall level from Whitelaw's *Epitome*. The average parish, south of the Liffey, housed 7,031 persons, mostly female, on 41.37 standard acres. North of the river, in a smaller aggregate of five parishes created to augment ancient St. Michan's, density average 8,135 adults and children on 52.76 acres per parish. Population densities north and south were 169.70 and 128.50 persons to an acre. Density per building averaged 12.30 persons on the south side of the river, and it was highest in the parishes of St. Michael and St. Luke. The least density per structure was at Christ Church, the area home to celibate professors from Trinity College. More typical was the

Table 5.2 No. XIV. Parish of Saint Anne

	Population			Houses	
Name of street, and c.	Males	Females	Totals	Inhabited	Waste
Lower Merion st. W.side	12	16	28	7	0
Upper Merion st. W.side	108	145	253	21	2
Lacy's-lane	27	41	63	4	0
Merion-row, N.side	28	31	59	7	3
St. Stephen's green, N.	139	213	352	31	2
Kings's-st. South,N.side	110	191	301	28	0
Lime-kiln-yard	7	5	12	3	0
Johnston's-place	13	27	40	6	0
William-street, E.side	127	153	280	29	2
Exchequer-st. S.side From William-street to Grafton-street	72	104	176	19	1
Wilson's-yard	3	7	15	3	0
Clarendon-street	211	306	517	53	3
Clarendon-market, in 5 Stalls	6	11	17	5	0
Clarendon-row	63	76	139	4	0
Chatham-row	25	27	52	3	1
Coppinger's-row	11	18	29	3	1
Grafton-street, E.side Entire; W.side, from Kings-street to Exchequer-street	438	497	935	92	4
Adami-court	37	43	80	8	0
Grafton or Spann's Lane	97	126	223	10	0
Tangier-land	18	20	38	3	0
Chatham-street	67	91	158	18	3
Pitt-street	41	48	89	13	0
Harry-street	23	30	53	7	0
Johnston's-court	51	49	100	8	4
Dawson-street	269	373	642	60	3
Duke-street	119	150	269	23	0
Anne-street	113	168	281	30	0
Molesworth-street	160	233	393	37	0
Frederick-street	110	169	279	35	3
Kildare-street	170	232	402	46	0
Schoolhouse-lane	36	63	99	4	0
Nassau-street, S.side	119	168	287	34	1
Nassau-lane	8	6	14	1	0
Leinster-street, S.side	65	85	150	13	0
Clare-street	82	141	223	26	1
Clare-lane	34	29	63	4	0
Park-st.E.side & S.side	47	65	112	11	2
Total	3071	4157	7228	711	36

density rate of 10.17 per dwelling in St. Anne's parish. Among the five north side parishes ancient St. Michan's was the most crowded with 12.46 persons per dwelling, and St. George's was the least compacted with 8.68 persons per dwelling. For all 21 parishes—a number which expanded and contracted over time—the average number of persons per house was 11.82.

It was in this setting of crowded hourses cheek-byjowl on narrow, dirty streets that children played; there, families raised their infants, and some parents saw them die from diseases spread by unavoidable contacts. Plagues occurred regularly, and tuberculosis was widespread. Within unhygienic rooms those little children who survived passed their days.

A closer focus on the impact of insalubrious conditions on the mortality of children amidst the teeming streets is possible by estimating the number of children in each parish, and then extrapolating from numerical sources the number of children who might have survived, *mutatis mutandis*. In Whitelaw's later years he witnessed the first modern-style attempt to conduct a census in Ireland, in 1821, and the first of a series of increasingly accurate censuses (Jordan 1997). The 1821 census (p. 26) lists the number of surviving children in each parish of "The County of the City of Dublin." In that year there were 24,149 children under the age of 5 years among a total population of 185,181 persons; they amounted to 13% of the whole. Two estimates of mortality among the young came from Sir William Wilde in 1843, and more recently from O Grada (O Grada 1991) who examined nineteenth century files at the rotunda maternity hospital which served the poorer districts of central Dublin. In both instances mortality among the young was estimated at 50%. This figure agrees with the findings of Edmund Halley and Sir William Petty in the previous century; it was a horrendous rate, one still evident as the nineteenth century matured, especially among the poor and among residents of industrial areas of the British Isles (Jordan 1993a, b).

Taking the proportion of the population ages 5 years and under from the 1821 census and applying it to the population of Dublin in 1798, Table 5.3 estimates the number of children 5 years and under in that year. The estimate of the number of young children is 4,817, and St. Peter's parish housed the largest group. Christ Church had the least, and they probably were the children of servants.

From the several estimates of mortality in the years under five it is apparent that the estimates in the first column represent one-half of the initial population. On that premise Table 5.3 lists in the second column double the number in the first column. That number is 9,634 children, and it estimates the scale of destruction wrought in the 1790s on the city of Dublin's juvenile population. That is not to say that there were ever circumstances in which none of the 9.634 little children would have died; rather, it sketches the gap between mortality and potential survival in an urban population as the eighteenth century drew to a close.

Finally, to return to the topic of quality of life; Dublin was a city combining Georgian grace in its more favored squares and streets and squalor in its crowded, noisome quarters. Some people made their way successfully; an example is Arthur

Table 5.3 Actual and potential survivors under age 5 years, 1798

Parish	Survivors 5 years and under survivors	Potential
St. James	92	184
St. Catherine	207	414
St. Luke	39	78
St. Nicholas without (the Walls)	90	180
St. Nicholas within	41	82
St. Audeon	143	286
St. Michael	30	60
St. John	84	168
St. Werburgh	151	302
Christ Church	5	10
St. Patrick	18	36
St. Bridget	355	710
St. Peter	689	1,378
St. Anne	419	838
St. Andrew	372	744
St. Mark	166	332
St. Paul	232	464
St. Michan	353	706
St. Mary	711	1,422
St. Thomas	382	764
St. George	238	476
Total	4,817	9,634

Guinness who, in 1798, oversaw a flourishing commercial venture at St. James' Gate providing wages and a proportionate degree of security and welfare to some of the residents of Dublin's teeming streets.

References

Berry, H. F. (1907). *The registers of the church of St. Michan, Dublin, 1636–1685.* Dublin: Parish Register Society of Dublin.

Butlin, R. A. (1965). The population of Dublin and the late seventeenth century. *Irish Geography, 5*, 51–66.

Butlin, R. A. (1977). Irish towns in the sixteenth and seventeenth centuries. In, *The development of the Irish town.* London: Croom Helm.

Empey, A. (2009). *The proctor's accounts of the Parish church of St. Werburgh, Dublin, 1481–1627.* Dublin: Four Courts.

Gillespie, R. (2004). *The vestry records of the parishes of St. Catherine and St. James, Dublin.* Dublin: Four Courts.

Jordan, T. E. (1993a). "L'Homme Moyen": Estimating the quality of life for British adults 1815–1914, an index. *Social Indicators Research, 29*, 183–203.

Jordan, T. E. (1993b). *The degeneracy crisis and victorian youth.* Albany: State University of New York Press.

Jordan, T. E. (1997). A century of Irish censuses. *New Hibernia Review, 2*, 94–114.

Jordan, T. E. (2006). *Gerard Boate's natural history of Ireland*. Lewiston: Mellen.
Jordan, T. E. (2010a). Quality of family life and mortality in seventeenth century Dublin. *Social Indicators Research, 98*, 251–263.
Jordan, T. E. (2010b). *Studies in the quality of life and human development in Ireland and Britain since the sixteenth century*. Lewiston: Mellen.
Jordan, T. E. (2010c). Quality of living conditions in eighteenth century Dublin: Whitelaw's survey, 1798. In *Studies in the quality of life and human development in Ireland and Britain since the sixteenth century*. Lewiston, NY: Mellen.
Mills, J. (1906). *The registers of St. John the Evangelist, Dublin, 1619–1699*. Dublin: The Parish Registers Society of Dublin.
Mills, J. (1911). *The registers of the Parish of St. Peter and St. Kevin 1699–1761*. Dublin: Parish Register Society.
Ni Mhurchadha, M. (2007). *The vestry records of the united parishes of finglas, st. Margaret's, Artane, and the ward, 1657–1758*. Dublin: Four Courts.
O Grada, C. (1991). Dublin's demography in the early nineteenth century: evidence from the Rotunda. *Population Studies, 45*, 43–54.
Parish Register Society of Dublin. (1908). *The registers of S. Catherine, Dublin,* 1636–1715. Dublin.
Wallace, W. J. R. (2011). *The vestry records of the parish of St. Bride, 1662–2741*. Dublin: Four Courts.

Chapter 6
Nineteenth Century Ireland

Within the United Kingdom Ireland's 32 counties in four provinces, Ulster, Leinster, Munster, and Connacht, held an anomalous position. In the sixteenth century, Henry VIII declared that his kingdom included Ireland. Elizabeth conducted ineffective campaigns against uprisings, and James VI and I settled his fellow Scots in Ireland's northeastern province, Ulster. There, Scottish Presbyterians displaced Gaelic Catholics and precipitated tensions still burning today. The nineteenth century's early decades saw Daniel O'Connell's efforts to repeal the earlier Act of Union, and his successful campaign for Catholic emancipation. The subsequent decades leading to the events of 1916 were plagued by British politicians' ambivalence about Ireland. It was viewed simultaneously as "the sister island"—to use nineteenth century idiom—and also as an alien place full of dangerous people.

With the 1801 Act of Union Ireland's politicians placed their fate in the hands of the legislature at Westminster reasoning that the influence of their MP's would be greater at the seat of power. That strategy did not work, and led to Daniel O'Connell's campaign for repeal of the Act of Union. However, Dublin Castle received fair spirited administrators from time to time. Two may be mentioned briefly; they were Thomas Drummond who died young, and Thomas A. Larcom who had a long and distinguished career. He went to Ireland to serve as an engineer in the Ordnance Survey and Larcom became an influential Commissioner for the census of 1841. He went on to serve as Under Secretary for Ireland at Dublin Castle having served on the Board of Works during the famine years (Jordan 2002, 2003). Improvement in Ireland's quality of life is evident across the nineteenth century due to a variety of factors. Larcom, and Drummond to a lesser extent, influenced governance positively through their integrity at Dublin Castle. Their conduct in office stands in contrast to the management of land across Ireland and the quality of life within which ordinary people labored in the face of land clearance and high rents.

This set of facts is relevant to mortality among Irish children because their situation was influenced by the self-serving practices of absentee landlords, and by the suspicions generated by Fenian bombers on the larger island. The condition of

T. E. Jordan, *Quality of Life and Mortality Among Children*,
SpringerBriefs in Well-Being and Quality of Life Research,
DOI: 10.1007/978-94-007-4390-8_6, © The Author(s) 2012

Ireland, unlike much of England and Wales, and Scotland, was pastoral, for the most part. Beyond Dublin and expanding Belfast there were few towns of any size other than Cork, Limerick, and Galway. The nonurban population was rural, poor, and lived in pitiful cottages, and city folk lived in no less appalling housing (Jordan 2011a, b). Table 6.1 lists the population of Ireland 1821–1891.

The rural economy in the nineteenth century was largely cash poor, and people relied on the fickle potato long after its failure in the late 1840s. Each summer saw a period of hunger before the new potato crop was lifted, so that hunger among children was inevitable. Resources in the form of medical care and supportive social institutions were slow to emerge (Geary 2004), and sick children died.

For example, in the famine year 1848 dysentery—today treated largely by rehydration—took the lives of James Early age 4 years, and his sister Bridget; their deaths occurred on 12 January in the workhouse at Navan, in County Meath. A few weeks later, Ann Monaghan, age six, died of an unspecified fever. She was one of 39 children under 8 years of age who died at Navan in early 1848 (Connell 2004).

The deaths in the Navan workhouse occurred in the famine years; however, their deaths from fever might have come about in any year because typhus had been endemic in Ireland for centuries. Transmitted by the bite of fleas and lice the disease was one of the complex of problems traceable to a lack of personal hygiene. Equally likely to generate fever was typhoid, but that disease was more a matter of drains—or the lack of them. In that regard conditions described by the rev. Mr. James Whitelaw of Dublin 1805 persisted for decades facilitating the spread of disease (Jordan 2011a, b).

Death among children may be construed at several levels between the grief of family members and, at the other extreme, an abstract, numerical resource. Whatever the idiom, children's mortality in nineteenth century Ireland occurred within society as a whole. A brief consideration of Ireland in the form of statistical data provides a background for a numerical analysis of death among the young. Table 6.1 from the 1891 census shows the radical change in population in the preceding decades. In 1821, there were 6.80 million people in Ireland, a number rising above 8.17 millions in the early 1840s but declining to 6.55 millions in the post-famine census of 1851. Munster and Ulster had the largest populations.

Across the troubled period 1841–1911 the greatest percentage of loss of families, i.e., more than 4%, occurred in the counties Queen's, Monaghan, Mayo, and Roscommon. Some increased in population, and they were led by Antrim, Dublin, and Kildare.

Figure 6.1 schematizes the trend of three social variables from 1831 to 1901; they are the number of families, the extent of literacy, and the course of wages. The data points plotted in Fig. 6.1 consist of 15 index numbers at intervals of 5 years. Each index number is the percentage of the relevant variable in 1901. As an example, wages in 1831 were about 18% of the criterion value in 1901.

Figure 6.1 shows that the number of families in Ireland fell sharply after the famine, and then declined at a less precipitate rate until 1901. Literacy among persons 5 years of age and above rose steadily across the century despite a trough

Table 6.1 Showing, by provinces, the total population of Ireland at each census period, 1821–1891

Census periods	Ireland	Province of				Census periods
		Leinster	Munster	Ulster	Connaught	
Persons						
1821[a]	6,801,827	1,757,492	1,935,612	1,998,494	1,110,229	1821
1831[a]	7,767,401	1,090,713	2,227,152	2,286,622	1,343,914	1831
1841[a]	8,175,124	1,972,731	2,396,161	2,386,373	1,418,859	1841
1851[a]	6,552,385	1,672,738	1,857,736	2,022,880	1,010,031	1851
1861[a]	[a]5,798,564	1,457,635	1,513,558	1,914,236	913,135	1861
1871[a]	5,412,377	1,339,451	1,393,485	1,833,228	846,213	1871
1881[a]	5,174,836	1,278,989	1,331,115	1,743,075	821,657	1881
1891[a]	4,701,750	1,187,760	1,172,402	1,619,814	724,774	1891
Males						
1821[a]	3,341,926	859,798	960,119	968,061	553,948	1821
1831[a]	3,794,880	927,877	1,093,411	1,113,094	660,498	1831
1841[a]	4,019,576	963,747	1,186,190	1,161,797	707,842	1841
1851[a]	3,190,630	813,537	904,979	976,312	495,802	1851
1861[a]	[a]2,836,977	715,005	744,682	923,255	454,035	1861
1871[a]	2,639,753	655,114	686,106	879,805	418,728	1871
1881[a]	2,533,277	630,038	659,901	826,224	407,021	1881
1891[a]	2,318,953	587,847	587,611	781,329	363,166	1891
Females						
1821[a]	3,459,901	897,694	975,493	1,030,433	556,281	1821
1831[a]	3,972,521	981,836	1,133,741	1,173,528	623,416	1831
1841[a]	4,155,548	1,009,984	1,209,971	1,224,576	711,017	1841
1851[a]	3,361,755	859,201	952,757	1,035,568	514,229	1851
1861[a]	[a]2,961,587	742,630	768,876	990,981	459,100	1861
1871[a]	2,772,624	684,337	707,379	954,423	427,485	1871
1881[a]	2,641,559	648,951	671,121	906,851	414,636	1881
1891[a]	2,385,797	599,913	584,791	838,485	362,608	1891

[a] Exclusive of 403 persons 393 males and 10 females—at sea on Census night—7th April, 1861
Note—The Census of 1821 is the first that affords a means of comparison with those of subsequent decades

at midcentury. On the other hand, wages rose steadily and peaked around 1871 before declining.

Table 6.1 and Fig. 6.1 are an abstraction of selected aspects of Ireland, and both provide a longitudinal view of progress in elements of quality of life. Beyond the scope of this empirical abstraction are major elements such as the famine—which set the framework for life in the era to be addressed in numerical terms here—emigration, the decline and rediscovery of the Irish language, and the land question. These events are touched on here as background, and they are auxiliary rather than central to the deaths of children in the analysis to be undertaken.

From Willis's 1845 survey of life in Dublin just before the famine I have calculated the loss of life among the children of 22 quite ordinary residents. The group excludes three men who reported no baptized children. The group covered a

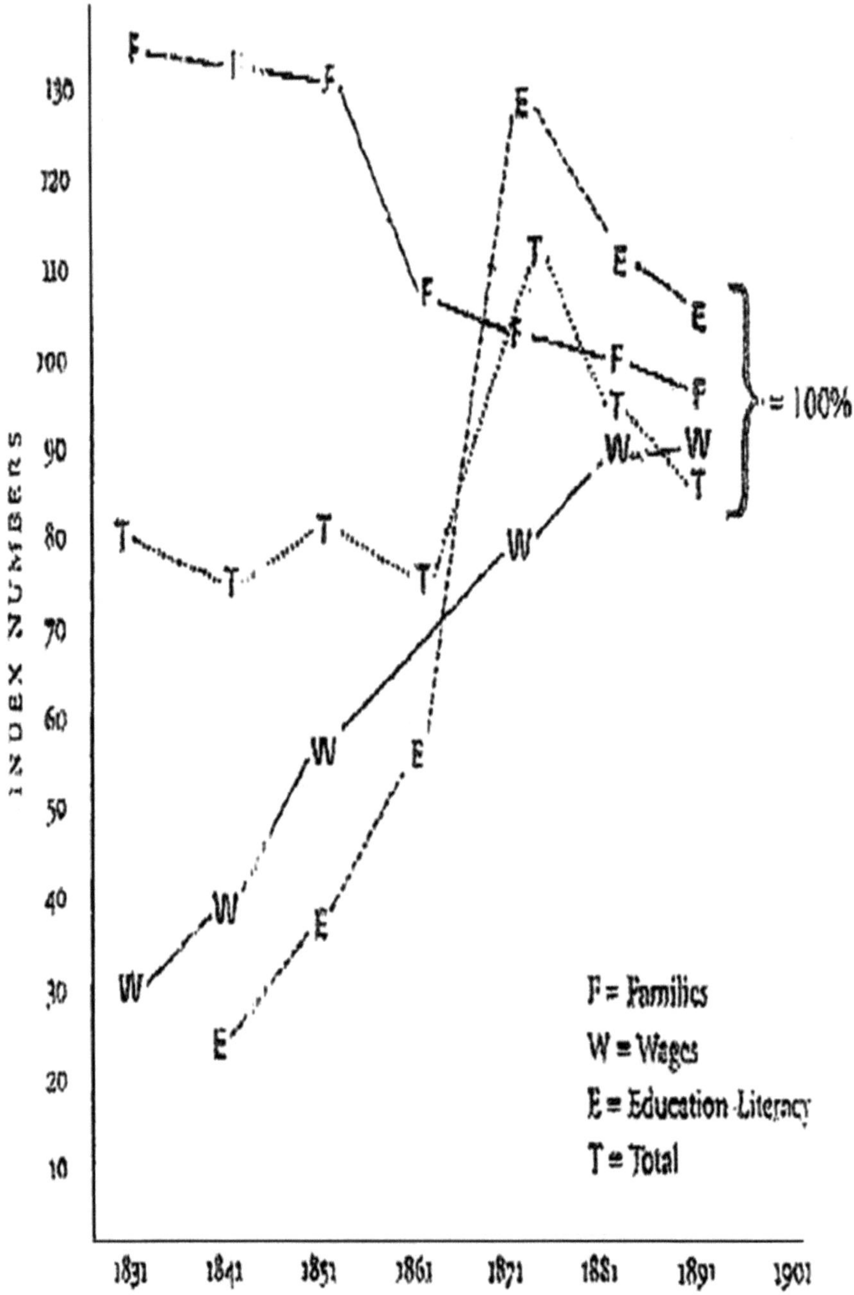

Fig. 6.1 Three domain indexes and total index (1901 = 100)

range of skilled occupations from carpenter to baker, with a range of ages from 25 to 52 years, and averaged 35 years. One man, a taylor from nearby Wicklow, was a bachelor; and a coach painter born in King's county was a widower.

Data on the children do not include age at death, but merely record the children "now living." The group of children recorded as baptized permits no inference about any children not baptized. As we have seen the average age of the men is in their thirties, and the age at marriage recorded by Willis was 23, with a range of 18–38 years. This suggests that the children who did not survive possibly were less than 10 years of age when they died. Among the male children of the 22 men who had children, 66 were baptized; their mortality I calculate to be 44%. Among 62 baptized females the number reported to have died was 32—which is 48%. When the genders are combined 128 baptisms were followed in later years by 69 deaths—46%, or almost one half.

Willis recorded background data on the 25 men considered here. Eleven were Dublin-born, and only one was born far away, a shoemaker from Limerick. Practically all the families lived in one room; one man, a lastmaker, lived in a cellar, and a printer's family lived in two rooms at a rent of 30 shillings a week. For the rest, rents ranged from one shilling and threepence (15d.) to three shillings (36d). "Wages when employed" averaged 22 shillings a week; however, only 10 men reported their employment to Willis as "constant." From Willis's 1845 survey we glimpse the context within which the deaths of children took place. The ratio of rent to unstable income was, on average, that of two shillings and a farthing (24.28d.) out of a weekly wage of 21 shillings. In addition to rent there were expenditures for food, clothing, and medicine, etc. for a family unit which I generalize as two adults and two children.

Death amongst the children of Dublin artisans seems predictable, broadly speaking; the typical family's quality of life came from a small and unstable income to support living in one room. Overcrowding placed family members at risk within their tiny living space; it was probably one of several in a building housing several sets of tenants. The unnamed lastmaker married at 18 a lass of 15. The cellar for which he paid two shillings a week sheltered the parents and a cumulative total of eight children, although that number probably was never attained since children died at various times. The highest paid artisan was a slater earning an unstable wage of 28 shillings per week. This family lived in two rooms and none of their children survived.

For the final 37 years of the nineteenth century the rate of mortality for all ages and both genders averaged, by my calculation, from the tables drawn up by Vaughan and Fitzpatrick (1978) 17.83 deaths per 1,000 persons. Mortality probably was highest among children born into the most disadvantaged families—given the associated squalor. In 1845 Willis calculated cumulative mortality "… amongst upward of 3,000 families of the working classes …" in Dublin. By the end of the first year of life cumulative mortality was 32.28%; by the end of the second year it had risen to 41.60%. By the third birthday 45.87 of the birth cohort had perished, and by age four the loss had risen to 49.35%. At age five 51.66% of children in Willis's set of 3,000 families were dead. Subsequently, the mortality rate continued to decline, but two-thirds (65.93%) of working class children were dead by age 20 years.

Willis took his data one more step by introducing a calculation of life expectancy—much of which came from the ancient parish of St. Michan which lies a little north of the river Liffey. Should a child reach the first birthday, Willis calculated that it might attain the age of 23.48 years. The optimum life expectancy, 30.21 years, was the potential for those young people still alive at age 14. Beyond age 14 life expectancy declined in linear fashion.

For children who survived the famine years, a period in which death was likely to come from the correlated malnutrition and lowered resistance to disease, there were health problems. Other symptoms were learning problems and susceptibility to infections. The social context within which Willis's findings emerged, namely a decade of improving wages and education, is evident in Fig. 6.2.

The Rotunda. A series of studies of the Dublin Hospital for Poor Lying-In Women by O Grada (1991, 1995) provides insight into infant mortality. Founded by Bartholomew Mosse in 1745 in Dublin's Northside The Rotunda, as it is known, provided a record of deliveries and the outcome for mothers and newborns. In the years 1830–1837 there were 16,645 deliveries and associated with them were 54.70 stillbirths per 1,000 births, and 8.80 child deaths per 1,000 live births. Maternal deaths were 10.60 per 1,000 births. Comparable data in London, according to O Grada, yielded rates of 7.50 and 9.20 maternal deaths per K (1,000) births. At the Rotunda about one half of maternal deaths were due to puerperal fever, one of the diseases of uncleanliness in hospitals.

For newborns at the Rotunda, O Grada concluded, the prospects for reaching age 5 years were about one-in-two, a probability which improved for those higher in the range of social classes—bearing in mind that the Rotunda's population was drawn largely from Dublin's poor. They resided in the northside's ancient parish of St. Michan, and in the parishes of SS. James, Catherine, Luke, Bride, Michael, and Nicholas.

When mother and child were released from the Rotunda they returned to the appalling conditions described by Whitelaw (1805) and Willis (1845). In Whitelaw's survey St. Michan's parish embraced 18,092 persons who lived 182.6 persons per acre. Such density of residents facilitated the spread of disease and contributed to the shortened life expectancy for little children. However, the Rotunda records provide evidence of a modest improvement in child development over the decades. In the last quarter of the nineteenth century the average birthweight was 3,250 gm., and in the early decades of the twentieth century the average birthweight rose modestly to 3,350 gm. Speculation suggests that the gain in birthweight was shared by preemies, a surmise supported by O Grada's identification of a reduction of 3% in the frequency of low birthweight infants. Current practice sets a threshold of 2,500 gm. (5 1/2 lb.) for a reasonable expectation of weight at birth. Of course, nineteenth century Dublin, like other centers of population, lacked today's armory of interventions for babies of low birthweight.

In the course of normal development children were likely to encounter an array of disease for which there were no specific remedies. Evaluation of symptoms evolved leading to separation of diphtheria and scarlet fever. In the era William Little published his monograph on cerebral palsy, and John H. Langdon-Down

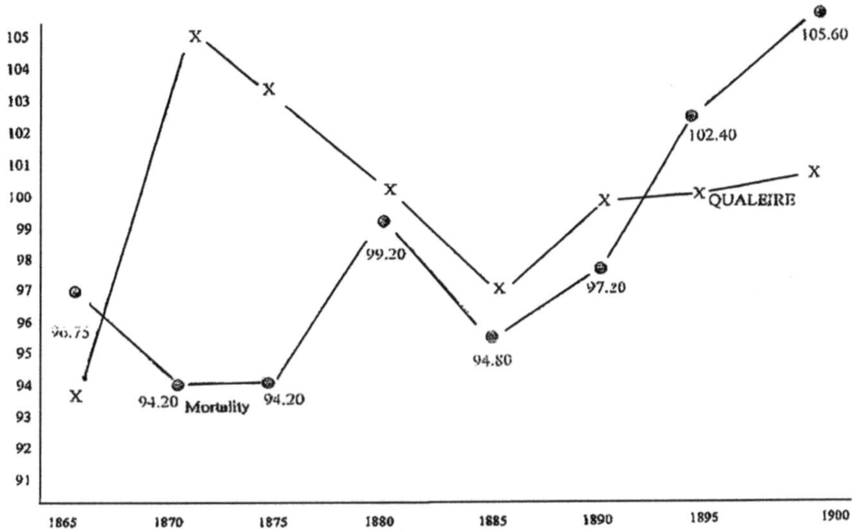

Fig. 6.2 QUALEIRE and infant mortality rate index numbers 1862–1902

mis-perceived—but in an eventually helpful way—the developmental disorder bearing his name (Jordan 2001). Dr. Lawson Tait introduced the appendectomy, and Queen Victoria accepted chloroform when delivering her son, Leopold, thereby popularizing anesthesia. In Dublin there were modest indicators of improvements, and ophthalmia was pioneered by Sir William Wilde.

6.1 Post-Famine Mortality

The last half-century of the Victorian era opened with the Medical Charities Act in 1851. One hundred and 63 poor law unions, the issue of the 1838 Irish poor law, sponsored 960 dispensaries which were served by 776 physicians (Geary 2004). Just before the famine, Thomas Willis repeated a call first formalized in 1812 for "… the better regulation and preservation of parish and other registries of births, baptisms, marriages, and burials …" Willis insisted that such a system "should be extended to Ireland" (noting that) "the importance of a well-regulated system cannot be too highly valued" (Willis 1845). However, two decades passed before Ireland installed the necessary procedures pursuant to laws passed in 1863 and 1864. It may be recalled that the 1838 poor law had generated the workhouses to which the starving had fled in the late 1840s.

For children in the post-famine years the gauntlet of biosocial hazards still had to be run; uterine health and fetal development inclined some babies to stillbirth or an early death. Those who survived infancy faced measles, chickenpox, and the other diseases of childhood. In the case of what we now refer to as strep throat there were sequelae which were not apparent, but which would appear as heart problems in later years. For children, like adults, there was always the risk of tuberculosis, a disease both infectious and fatal in the long run.

Our grasp of death among children in the post-famine era is restricted as a national aggregate by the comparatively late date at which registration of births and deaths became obligatory—1864.

6.2 A Descriptive Estimate

The tool used here to explore the social matrix within which young Irish children died is the QUALEIRE index of quality of life (Jordan 2000). Composed of 14 variables in four domains this index, as with the VICQUAL index in the previous chapter, provides a longitudinal, or time, series of information estimating the condition of the general population of Ireland. Given the source, index numbers can be used to develop a schematic representation of the connection between QUALEIRE index numbers and mortality among children under 1 year in the last half of the nineteenth century.

The dependent measure is the incidence of mortality per 1,000 live births expressed here as 5 year averages and indexed to the rate in 1902. Civil registration began in Ireland after passage of laws in 1863 and 1864, so that the data set employed here covers four decades (Mitchell 1971). This apparent limitation is offset to a degree by the observation that, "… the infant mortality rate … (is) an important and significant indicator … the scale of infant mortality has important consequences" (Lee 1991)—the canary in the coal mine, as it were.

Figure 6.3 illustrates the course of QUALEIRE index numbers from 1862 to 1902. The number of observations in Fig. 6.3 for each of the two variables is eight, a number too low to correlate variables. Figure 6.4 presents average quinary data centered on the years 1865, 1870 … 1900. The numbers next to the closed circles are the quinary death rates of infants per 1,000 live births. The series of connected "X" symbols are the quinary sets of QUALEIRE index numbers. The technique of analysis is inspection of the two profiles of data to identify trends across time in which, for example, rising QUALEIRE index numbers indicative of an improving quality of life anticipate declining mortality rates. A perfect relationship would be evident in two straight lines, one rising and one lagged across the years, and meeting in the criterion year 1902. Matching index numbers in the two profiles is not causally relevant.

For the first decade rising and falling quality of life is inversely paralleled by falling and then declining mortality for infants under 1 year. Across the last decade deaths rose more sharply than the quality of life rates. From 1880 to 1890 the lines are roughly parallel. The overall impression is that the indexed mortality rate among children and the estimated quality of life connect only a little better than chance. Mortality seems to have its own dynamic amid the social context.

However, aggregation of the QUALEIRE source domains might hide more discriminating relationships with mortality among Irish children in the Victorian era. To examine that possibility the next four figures connect three subdomains—

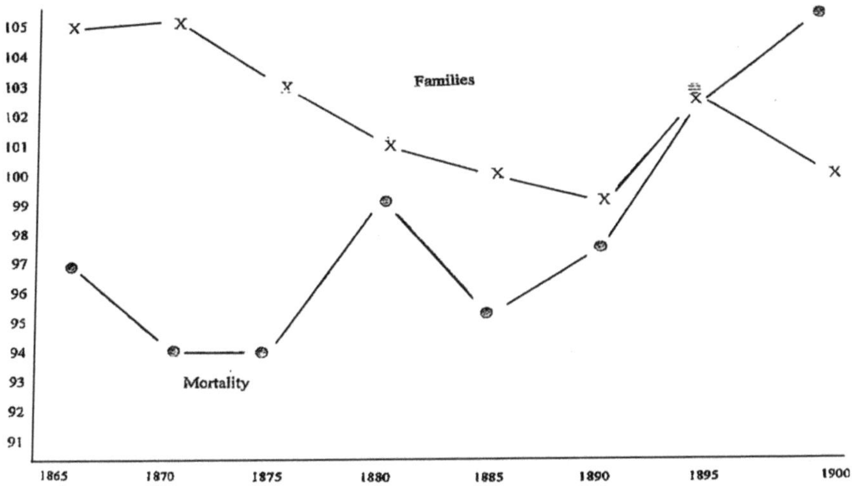

Fig. 6.3 QUALEIRE *families* and infant mortality rate index numbers, 1864–1902

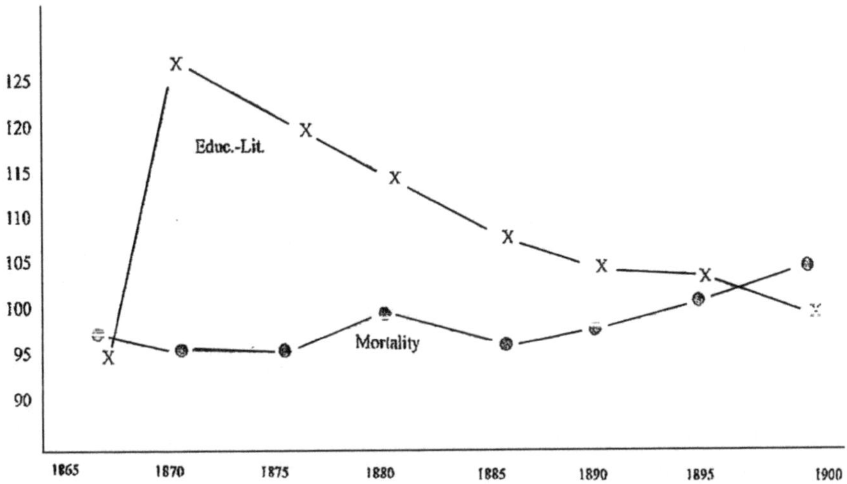

Fig. 6.4 QUALEIRE *education-literacy* and infant mortality rate index numbers, 1864–1902

Families, Education and Literacy, and Wages with the mortality rate. It should be noted that the horizontal axis representing dates in each figure is identical, but the vertical axis varies in accordance with the range of index numbers which varies from schema to schema.

Families. This component of the QUALEIRE index consists of four elements: birth rate per 1,000 of the population, the number of families, the number of persons per family, and mortality per 1,000 births. These items were taken from the censuses conducted at intervals of 10 years (Jordan 1997, 1998). It is evident

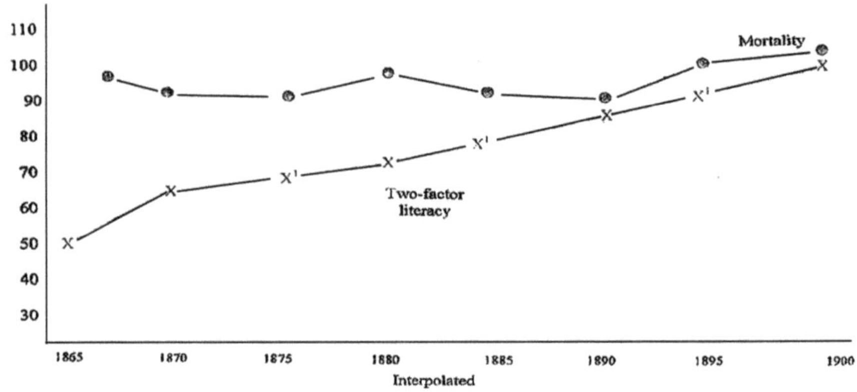

Fig. 6.5 Two-factor QUALEIRE *education-literacy* and infant mortality rate index numbers, 1864–1902

that the last item in the series, mortality, is one-fourth of the family component, posing the risk of confounding the model, and should be kept in mind when considering the family mortality relationship.

In Fig. 6.5 the two lines are contradictory after 1865 but become closer by 1880 being separated by only a few points. In 1890 the two indexes are quite close, and 5 years later they are still closer. More focally, the 5 years after 1890 trend in the same direction implying that child mortality rose toward the criterion rate in 1902, while the quality of families also rose. After 1895 the two trend lines diverge sharply; the numerical quality of families rose, while mortality declined. The general observation is that the numerical account of families and the rate of children's mortality occasionally can be connected as trend lines, but in most of the 5 year intervals across the last four decades of the nineteenth century they are quite independent.

Education and Literacy. The four elements in this portion of the QUALEIRE index of quality of life are: female illiteracy, school enrollments, attendance at school, and letters delivered. School enrollments are available since 1841, and it may be noted that Ireland received its national system of elementary schools several decades before England and Wales. Female illiteracy was not recorded until 1871, and attendance data were first recorded in 1861. The consequence is that the complex addressed here can be viewed as an evolving index of quality of life. Three elements were present in 1861, and all four were available by 1871. Education and literacy improved across the nineteenth century as a falling population and increasing use of the postal system itself an index of literacy flourished. Across the decades addressed here the four factor Education—Literacy complex changed steadily, and child mortality index numbers fluctuated only modestly. Generally speaking, the Education—Literacy complex moved towards the 1902 criterion values while child mortality rose and fell. However, across the four decades as a whole, mortality remained a largely autonomous process.

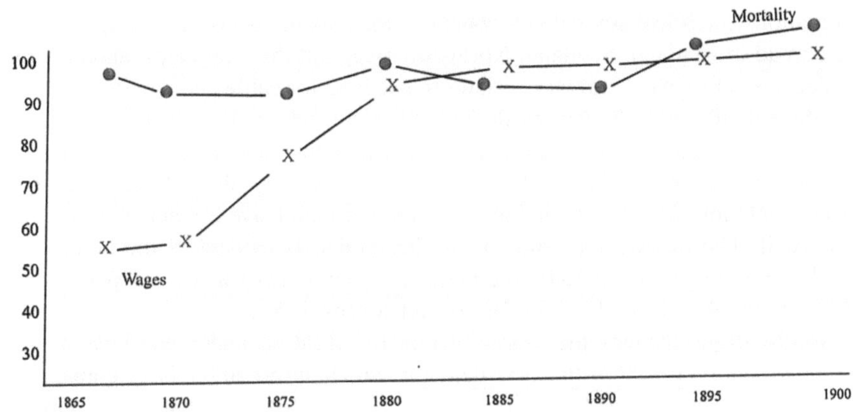

Fig. 6.6 QUALEIRE *wages* and infant mortality rate index numbers, 1864–1902

An alternative to use of four elements is given in 6.6. There two elements, school enrollment and letters delivered, are plotted against mortality. In the first 10 years sharply rising literacy is matched by mildly declining mortality index numbers. For the decade, 1880–1890 the lines are reciprocal, one rising while the other, child mortality, falls. Note the interpolation for 1875, 1885, and 1895. Use of the two-factor antecedent does not seem to improve the connection between the Education—Literacy component of quality of life and infant mortality.

Wages. Wage data from nineteenth century Ireland do not appear to have been gathered systematically across the 32 counties until Bowley's (1900) account. O Grada (1994) presented wages in pennies per week in a series in which wages doubled between 1850 and 1893. There was a one-time survey by the Poor Law Commissioners in 1870. In this study four accounts of wages across the period of interest are employed; the longest series is from Cork and was drawn from laborers. Wages from two series are a little less complete; they also are from agricultural laborers. A briefer series of wage data ending in 1851 was taken from Masons. See Jordan (2000).

Figure 6.6 shows mortality index numbers and combined wage data from laborers, after 1831, and at intervals of a decade. Mortality for children under 1 year was fairly consistent across the era, while laborers' wages rose dramatically. In 1831 laborers earned about one-half of the wages they received at the end of the century, and the rate of increase was most rapid before 1880. There seems no obvious connection between laborers' wages and rates of mortality; the former was dynamic while the latter began and ended the era having fluctuated only a little.

Nineteenth century Ireland experienced a great number of changes; the population prior to the mid-1840s expanded rapidly, only to fall at mid-century. The major impact on the people of Ireland was the collapse of the rural population's monodiet of the potato; this root vegetable had failed in several countries and then failed catastrophically in Ireland. This event may be studied elsewhere,for example, Woodham–Smith (1962). A major process after the period of famine was emigration which had several components. One was the decision to seek a better life abroad in England, Scotland, North America, and the Antipodes; another was the decision of managers of large estates to use land for cattle and its products, and to reduce land's costs by tearing down habitations subject to valuation and so to taxes. In such cases tenants were evicted, and in some cases their passage money to a destination set by the landlord's agent was the only alternative. Of course, some people migrated to population centers rather than leave Ireland, choosing the lesser evil. The devastation wrought by the famine is evident in the number of people who emigrated. In 1845, the number of emigrants was 81,177 persons; in 1849, the number was 231,626 (Carrier and Jeffrey 1953).

Amidst these changes the mortality rate for children under one year of age remained static. In 1864, the first date for which information is available, the mortality rate was 98 deaths per 1,000 births; it peaked in 1880 at 112 deaths. In the final years of the nineteenth century the mortality rates were high. For the last 5 years of the waning century the annual death rates averaged 105.60 deaths. As the new century opened, the mortality rate in 1902 was 100 deaths per 1,000 births.

Ideally, mortality data would exist at the level of each census unit, and by gender and age. Such information would be analyzed in a multivariate design, but such is not the case. On the other hand, the QUALEIRE estimate of the quality of life seems a fairly satisfactory estimate of Ireland's quality of life over several decades. It is apparent that Ireland improved in several aspects of quality of life, but improvement in infant mortality does not appear to have been one of them.

This exercise in numerical observation and deduction is better than mere conjecture. In the empirical idiom, infant mortality in nineteenth century Ireland emerges indeterminate, with occasional brief periods when social change relates to rates of mortality, but such speculations resist generalization.

6.3 Correlations

In this second analysis of QUALEIRE index numbers and child mortality rates per 1,000 (K) live births, the focus is closer than the graphic displays presented in Figs. 6.2, 6.3, 6.4, 6.5, 6.6. That is, QUALEIRE index numbers are employed in annual form, and are analyzed as the full index numbers, plus three subdomain index numbers (see Table 6.2) for a total of four correlations. The number of annual index numbers is 38 covering the years 1864–1901. Table 6.3 reports two-tailed r correlations.

Limitations of the data are: the quality of the Victorian mortality data (Mitchell and Deane 1971); the fusing of male and female data; the comparatively brief length of time covered—legislation for formal recording of vital information did not begin in Ireland until 1864, and earliest years were in the traumatic post-famine era; statistics are extant only for children born alive who died before their fifth birthday. Despite these limitation efforts at numerical analysis are better than speculation and anecdote.

Table 6.2 Index numbers of 12 QUALEIRE components in three domains (1901 = 100)

Variables	1861	1871	1881	1891	1901
Domain: Families					
Birthrate	106	123	108	101	100
Mortality	84	83	89	93	100
Persons/family	102	101	101	100	100
Families (millions)	174	116	108	102	100
Domain: Education and literacy					
Female illiteracy	–	223	172	132	100
School enrollment	42	59	65	76	100
Attend.≤100 days	82	145	123	105	100
Letters delivered	59	71	88	100	
Domain: Wages					
Cork city-laborers	–	90	97	97	100
Agriculture	71	78	90	100	–
Masons	18	–	–	100	–
Limerick-agriculture	75	92	100	–	–

Table 6.3 QUALEIRE means, and correlations (r) between annual QUALEIRE index numbers and annual infant mortality data, 1864–1901

	QUALEIRE *total*	QUALEIRE *families*	QUALEIRE *educ.–Lit.*	QUALEIRE *wages*
M	102.06	101.80	105.08	82.93
r	−0.03	−0.40	0.32	0.41
p	0.88	0.01	0.05	0.01

Across the last four decades of the nineteenth century in Ireland the quality of life as estimated by the QUALEIRE index generally rose. Among the four predictors in Table 6.3 the trend of the first three is for quality of life to increase as child mortality declined. In contract, the fourth element was positive but not statistically significant. More particularly, the full QUALEIRE index also was significantly related to mortality; the lack of a significant correlation may be traceable to a suppressor effect of the Wages component; see Table 6.2.

On the other hand, the variable, Families, composed of four elements was a useful predictor of child mortality ($p = 0.01$), as was the four-variable domain, Education—Literacy ($p = 0.05$). Those two factors help decipher the course of children's mortality across the four final decades of the nineteenth century. The array of eight elements suggests a social complex within which Ireland's youngest children lived and died at annual rate across the last four decades of 98.03 deaths per 1,000 live births; it may be recalled that the highest rates came as the nineteenth century blended into the twentieth century. The reality of high mortality rates appears understandable to a modest degree through use of the QUALEIRE index of quality of life; however, there remain residual, as yet unidentified, factors in Victorian Ireland which remain to be explicated across the final four decades.

References

Bowley, A. L. (1900). *Wages in the United Kingdom in the nineteenth century*. Cambridge: Cambridge University Press.
Carrier, N. H., & Jeffery, J. R. (1953). *External migration: A study of the available statistics*. London: General Register Office.
Connell, P. (2004). *The land and the people of county Meath, 1750–1850*. Dublin: Four Courts.
Geary, L. M. (2004). *Medicine and charity in Ireland, 1718–1851*. Dublin: University College Press.
Jordan, T. E. (1997). A century of Irish censuses. *New Hibernia Review, 2*, 94–114.
Jordan, T. E. (1998). *The census of Ireland, 1821–1911*. Lewiston: Mellen. Three volumes.
Jordan, T. E. (2000). The quality of life in Victorian Ireland, 1831–1901. *New Hibernia Review, 4*, 103–121.
Jordan, T. E. (2001). Quality of life, hegemony, and social change in rural Ireland. In: W. B. Jones (Ed.), *A landlord who tried to do his duty. Social Indicators Research, 55*, 199–221.
Jordan, T. E. (2002). *An imaginative empiricist: Thomas Aiskew Iarcom* (1801–1879) *and Victorian Ireland*. Lewiston, NY: Mellen.
Jordan, T. E. (2003). Two Thomases: Dublin Castle and the quality of life in Victorian Ireland. *Social Indicators Research, 64*, 257–291.
Jordan, T. E. (2011a). Whitelaw's essay on the population of Dublin (1805): A window on eighteenth century housing. *New Hibernia Review, 15*, 9–18.
Jordan, T. E. (2011b). Whitelaw's essay on the population of Dublin (1805): A window on late eighteenth century housing. *New Hibernia Review, 25*, 136–145.
Lee, C. H. (1991). Regional inequalities in infant mortality in Britain, 1861–1971: Patterns and hypotheses. *Population Studies, 45*, 55–65.
Mitchell, B. R., & Deane, P. (1971). *Abstract of British historical statistics*. Cambridge: Cambridge University Press.
Mitchell, B. R. (1971). *British historical statistics*. Cambridge: Cambridge University Press.
O Grada, C. (1991). Dublin's demography in the early nineteenth century: Evidence from the rotunda. *Population Studies, 45*, 43–54.
O Grada, C. (1994). *Ireland: A new economic history, 1780–1939*. Oxford: Claredon.
O Grada, C. (1995). The Rotunda hospital and the people of Dublin, 1745–1995. In Browne, E. (Ed.), *Masters, midwives, and ladies in waiting*. Dublin.
Vaughan, W. E., & Fitzpatrick, A. J. (1978). *Irish historical statistics, population, 1821–1971*. Dublin: Dublin Royal Irish Academy.
Whitelaw, J. (1805). *An essay on the population of Dublin*. Dublin: Dublin Graisberry and Campbell.
Willis, T. (1845). *Facts conected with the social and sanitary condition of the working classes in dublin*. Dublin: O'Gorman.
Woodham-Smith, C. (1962). *The great hunger*. New York: Harper and Rowe.

Chapter 7
Mortality Among Children

Death among children tends to be ignored by those who study child development. The obvious reason is that death is a denial of life—the essence of development. Death is rare today among children and so it is not apparent in the list of developmental challenges. On the other hand, the death of children can be approached as a criterion of development with a negative valence. In that formulation child mortality can be formulated in a dichotomous fashion; it becomes one-half of a criterion in research on populations and samples which is formulated as 1/0. The 1/represents living and the /0 represents dead subjects. or vice versa.

The topic arises in demographic studies and inquiries into vital statistics. There are rare conditions around which philanthropies have coalesced to generate funds for research; an example is the complex surrounding the unanticipated death of infants.

In contrast, child development before the twentieth century encounters mortality as an inescapable element in the life cycle, especially for the very young. It acquires further value because it played a role in the dynamics of cities whose population growth tended to stagnate, or even recede. As we have seen, Dublin in the early modern period recorded more deaths than births, a situation compounded by high rates of mortality among those born alive. Populations' life expectancies were lowered numerically by early deaths, although calculations of life expectancy based on an age after the slaughter, e.g., at age 5 years, give a more optimistic view. In the case of seventeenth century Dublin, in-migration from the hinterlands and the larger island across the Irish Sea account for the increasing population.

For people who survived the risk of an early death there was the prospect of family formation, rearing children, and the prospect of seeing their children's children grow toward maturity. That prospect was compromised by the early death of their own children, and that of their grandchildren. Also, there was the fact of their own early deaths. Life tables in the seventeenth and eighteenth century, e.g., the work of William Petty and John Graunt, and Thomas Short in the eighteenth century, indicate that the risk of death rose sharply in middle age for most folk.

T. E. Jordan, *Quality of Life and Mortality Among Children*,
SpringerBriefs in Well-Being and Quality of Life Research,
DOI: 10.1007/978-94-007-4390-8_7,

Quality of life. There arises the matter of strategy when examining life in eras before our own. A tool which has proved valuable is the concept, quality of life. Open to many operational forms, this idea can shed light on the circumstances within which children's deaths occurred. For the early modern period, quality of life may be inferred cautiously from entries in diaries and public materials. However, inferences from diaries and parish registers are minute; they may only illuminate an incident such as the of an abandoned baby, or a tussle between privileged men over a church seat prized for its proximity to the preacher, or further away but less exposed to draughts. Similarly, the exact place of interment within the church may reveal a social standing extrapolated into the nether world.

The presumption in this work has been that an increasing quality of life is associated with declining mortality. For the nineteenth century and later there are numerical sources on a greater scale from which indicants (rather than measures) can be derived. For the English-speaking world there are the censuses of England and Wales, and Ireland; they have been drawn on here to examine mortality data. Ireland's official record keeping on vital statistics began later, and so is less informative.

There are choices about where, when, and how to examine mortality in an era before our own. They generate choices which are subjective, while others are objective—in the sense that they are numeric in their data language. Broader than these matters of methodology is the continuity we find across centuries as families face the loss of a child. Mourning is a human trait, and it conveys in its records the continuity of the human experience across the centuries.

MIX
Papier aus verantwortungsvollen Quellen
Paper from responsible sources
FSC® C105338

If you have any concerns about our products, you can contact us on
ProductSafety@springernature.com

In case Publisher is established outside the EU, the EU authorized representative is:
Springer Nature Customer Service Center GmbH
Europaplatz 3, 69115 Heidelberg, Germany

Printed by Libri Plureos GmbH
in Hamburg, Germany